MW01614962

Why Can't I Lose Weight?
The Secrets To Successful Permanent Weight Loss

By Nicole Gilles, RD, CDE, CSR
Dietitian and Health Coach

Why Can't I Lose Weight?
The Secrets To Successful Permanent Weight Loss

© 2017 by Nicole Gilles. All rights reserved.

No part of this book may be reproduced, scanned, or distributed in any printed, mechanical or electronic form (including photocopying) without prior written permission from the author.

ISBN 978-1-943784-87-5
ISBN 978-1-946208-12-5

Disclaimer: The ideas and concepts presented in this book are intended to be for informational and educational purposes only, and are not intended to diagnose, cure, treat, or prevent any disease.

The concepts in this book are general recommendations and are not intended to be used as a substitute or replacement for professional medical advice or dietitian services. Readers are recommended to do their own research and make decisions in partnership with their personal medical provider.

The author and publisher claim no responsibility for any adverse effects, loss, or damage caused directly or indirectly as a result of the implementation, interpretation or application of any of the content or material in this book.

Also note that while the client stories in this book are real, their names have been altered to protect their privacy.

DEDICATION

This book is dedicated to all of you that have tried every diet out there, only to end up heavier than before. To all my past, present, and future clients, rest assured that this is not your fault and you are not broken. Please know that there is hope, and that the information on the forthcoming pages has helped thousands of people achieve a happier life and a healthier weight.

In order for this information to work, you will have to stop dieting and over-restricting food. I hope this book brings you peace and comfort in knowing that you are not alone - and you can do it!

I also dedicate this book to my family. To my husband and best friend, Jason, who supports me and my journey in helping others. To my beautiful children, Laila, and Colton, who are constant reminders of happiness and health. They listen to their bodies, and remind me to listen to mine. To my parents and sister, who have been with me on this journey and have encouraged me to keep going.

To my best friends, colleagues, and clients. To Britteny, Alice, and Kimberley, who believe in me when I lose sight. Thank you to everyone in my life who has shared their story with me, and allowed me to help when needed, (and who have helped me when I was in need).

Most of all, I thank God for the gift He has shared with me. I will share it with great responsibility each day.

-Nicole

INTRODUCTION

Hi, there! Thank you for reaching out. Are you ready to make a change and try something new? Maybe you've tried all those popular diets out there: No Carbs, No Fats, Cabbage Soup, diet pills – but nothing works. Not even the "heart healthy diet" your doctor gave you is changing things. You've even started counting your calories, but still can't get the weight off (and now you feel even worse). Maybe you started skipping meals to lose weight, but that didn't work either.

So if you have tried all this, then what else is left? First of all, have hope. You are not alone in your quest for a healthy weight. The information we have been using to lose weight hasn't been effective, because it wasn't the whole story. Not only was critical information left out - life altering parts - but some of the information we have been told is just plain wrong. This is a vital reason why we can cut calories, exercise our lives away, and still not lose weight.

Let me be the first to apologize for this. As a Registered Dietitian and Medical Professional, I was taught these same principles in obtaining my Bachelor's Degree. The problem is, not all of the principles have the clinical research to back them up. So, there is little (or no) proof to determine that these previous recommendations work. Many principles have been based on theories. Fortunately, new studies are being completed every day. The latest studies may stun you, as they did me.

In a nut shell, there is so much more to weight loss than just total calorie intake and expenditure. Weight loss is more connected with the types and quality of calories we consume, as well as our hormone levels. You may need to add or eliminate foods based on your symptoms, and we will delve into that in the coming chapters.

One of the most important things I can tell you that will help with weight loss, is to be open-minded. Be open to new truths. And be willing to put into practice many things which may seem contrary to what you have learned thus far about having a healthy body.

The truth begins now...

WHAT ARE CLIENTS SAYING ABOUT THIS INFORMATION?

"After having four babies in five years, I wanted my energy and body back. I tried counting calories, but felt awful. After speaking with Nicole, I realized why my way wasn't working. She outlined a personalized plan for me and led me every step of the way. Not only did I lose weight, but I learned how to eat healthy for myself and my family."
                    -S.M. (Six-figure earning entrepreneur)

"I have struggled with my weight since my first child was born in 2006. Being a working mom, I had no idea how to balance it all with fitness and eating well. Nicole has taught me the importance of prioritizing myself, so I can be the best I can be. Nicole is the epitome of motivation and a wealth of knowledge."
                    -B.E. (Personal Trainer)

"After suffering with high blood sugar for over 20 years, I didn't think there was anything I could do to change my situation. After just a few months of working with Nicole, my doctor decreased my medication treatment plan, and I feel so much better."
                    -D.S. (Professional Truck Driver)

"I have been seeing Nicole for over three years now. I was referred by my kidney doctor, because my weight was causing me to lose function of my kidney transplant. Over the years, Nicole has been incredibly patient with me - and encouraged me to take baby steps. I am back at my high school weight and my transplant is stable. Thanks, Nicole!"
                    -K.B. (Dedicated Mother and Wife)

"With respect to weight loss, I believe it helps take stress off the body in so many ways - physically, metabolically, emotionally, socially, and mentally. Nicole provides the skills and motivation to guide people to a healthier weight."

-Robert C., M.D. (Nephrology Specialist)

"She combines expertise with passion to not only empathize with those she serves, but to motivate them to bring about lasting change. There are few persons I can think of whose compassion and knowledge transmit into action, like Nicole. Whatever your goals, she can help you meet and exceed them."

-A.V. (RN, BSN, CNN, PHN)

"I began working with Nicole to lose weight for my daughter's wedding. Since I can remember, I secretly considered my self-worth by the number on the scale. During our telephone sessions, I learned to eat for nutrition only! I learned to focus on who I am as a person and how to care for myself in a healthy way. I learned that food is not an evil source trying to steal my value, but it's a tool to maintain strength and stamina to be happy and healthy..."

-B.E. (RN)

TABLE OF CONTENTS

TABLE OF CONTENTS

Reading Guide: Although you may be eager to skip ahead to a certain chapter, I would like to remind you that the body works together as a system. If one part is off, it can throw the whole system off. Each and every chapter is equally important. Missing information in a chapter can be the difference between losing weight and not, even if you don't think it is connected. The truth is, it's all related. The head bone is connected to the neck bone, the neck bone is connected to the back bone. Remember, this book was written for you. You deserve to soak up all the information possible to help you finally get to that healthy weight that you deserve, and stay there. Please know that you are worth it; that you deserve to be fit, happy, and healthy; that you are worth every second you dedicate to yourself and your personal growth. The world would not be the same without you. There is no one else in the world that can take your place. This world needs you and your contributions.

That is why you are here.

PART I
NOURISH YOUR MIND

Chapter 1
Open Your Mind To The Fact That Anything Is Possible

Let me introduce you to Shelly. You may relate to her, and understand exactly what she went through. Shelly - a friend of a friend - called me up one day and said, "I don't know what you did to help my friend, but I need your help!"

I could tell Shelly had been crying, and asked her to share with me how she thought I could help. With a soft, wavering voice, she started to tell me how she had five small children, and lately she had been feeling so tired and cranky that she couldn't keep up with her own life. She use to be happy and energized. She use to laugh, and loved spending time with her family. But now, she could barely drag herself out of bed, let alone care for her family. Feeling desperate and alone, she reached out to her long-time friend, Breanna.

One day, while sitting in a coffee shop waiting for Breanna to arrive, Shelly began reflecting on her life. She realized she really didn't know what had happened. It was like one day she looked in the mirror and didn't recognize herself. How did she become this tired and frustrated person? She often found herself yelling at her kids, and distancing herself from her husband.

Shelly thought, "Who am I? I never used to be like this." It was like someone had removed her batteries, but still expected her to keep moving. "And where did all this weight come from?" she wondered.

Shelly had tried all those fad diets, but nothing was bearable. She wanted so desperately to get rid of the extra weight that was slowing her down and making her miserable, but it seemed like the harder she tried, the worse things got. And the more she restricted food and worked out, the more weight she gained. Shelly was ready to throw in the towel. After all, if she tried this hard and nothing worked, then maybe this was just the way things were going to be. Maybe she was broken.

Shelly thought that her friend was going to sympathize with her. After all, Breanna had a few kids and had gained weight, too. Maybe having a family or a successful career meant that you have to sacrifice your body and your happiness. Maybe in order to have other pleasures in life, you have to let go of your own joy.

When Breanna walked into the coffee shop, Shelly was shocked to find that her friend looked amazing! Her skin was glowing, and she seemed relaxed, happy and energized. Instead of coffee, Breanna actually ordered a decaf tea. Shelly couldn't believe it. Breanna was her long-time coffee buddy. How could she survive without the energizing pick me up of coffee?

As the two friends sat by the window at the coffee shop, Shelly began sharing her struggles. Desperate to feel better, she asked Breanna, "What have you been doing? You look like you just got back from a vacation - so happy and healthy."

Breanna said that she used to feel the same way that Shelly was feeling. She had tried everything to lose weight and feel better. She gave up soda and tried all those popular diets, but nothing worked and she felt awful. She, too, was ready to give up. Until she met me, Nicole Gilles.

Breanna and I went to church together. She had seen me before, during, and after my pregnancy. I was *not* that cute little pregnant lady. Being 5'2" - and my husband being 6'3" - I grow

8-pound babies. Just before delivering my daughter, someone asked me if I was having twins (please don't ever ask a pregnant woman if she is having twins).

After delivering, I made it a priority to get back to my normal food and fitness routine. I wanted to be the best I could be, and I knew that carrying extra weight would slow me down (and weigh down my spirit). I was quickly able to get back into those pre-pregnancy clothes, and I began feeling so energized I could start running races again.

Breanna knew I was a Registered Dietitian, and had seen that it was possible to get one's life and body back after starting a family. So after church one day, she pulled me aside and said, "I want to feel good again. I will do whatever you say for three months and see what happens. Will you help me?"

Naturally, I said yes, and together we created a plan for her with food that she liked and portions that helped her feel satisfied. After just a week, she was amazed at how much better she felt. She had less frustration, more energy and joy, and was already starting to shed pounds. She couldn't believe it! After years of over-restricting food and killing herself at the gym - which didn't help her lose a pound - she was finally beginning to lose weight eating food she actually liked.

As she sipped her coffee, Shelly was amazed at Breanna's story. As she was listening, she found herself thinking that if Nicole could help Breanna, maybe she could find help with her, too.

That very day, Shelly went home and called me. We dove right in and developed a personalized plan based on the food she enjoyed, her imbalanced hormone levels, and the symptoms she was having. After just a week, she was less bloated, more energized, and less moody.

Shelly and I continued to work together over the next few weeks. We adjusted her intake as needed, based on what her body was telling her.

On some days, your body requests more fuel, or food, and other days it needs less. This often depends on how active you are. If you are sitting at your computer all day, you probably don't require as much fuel as chasing after three kids on a weekend.

During her time with me, Shelly learned how to boost her calorie burning, listen to her body's needs, and care for her own emotional needs. After 12 weeks, Shelly was down 20 pounds. She had plenty of energy to keep up with her children, and found herself laughing and actually playing with them again. Her husband couldn't believe the change. He was so relieved to have his wife back that he wanted to get on the program, too.

Over the years, I have referred to Shelly and her husband as my "Power Couple." Together, they lost over 50 pounds - despite having a large family and running their own businesses. I realized that if they were able to overcome all their obstacles and find success, anyone could.

Feeling inspired? Would you like to know the secret? Losing weight is not just about the calories. If it was that easy, 70 percent of Americans would not be overweight. And the crazy thing is, the inability to lose weight is not for lack of trying.

The weight loss industry is worth billions of dollars, spent by people "trying." But trying is frustrating when you end up not being able to shed those unwanted pounds for good.

Would you like to stop trying and start seeing success? I have helped thousands of people – from children to the elderly – shed the extra pounds, reverse certain diseases, and start living the life they long for (with the energy to sustain it!). Together we can make the changes that bring about the positive results you've been hoping for. Ready?

Let's get started now!

Chapter 2
It's All About Mindset – Believe and You Will Achieve

When an opportunity presents itself – even before we decide how to move forward – we very often think about how it will end for us; we predetermine the outcome with our emotions. Let's say I ask you to go for a walk tomorrow at 7:00 p.m. Before you even think about what you have going on tomorrow at 7:00 p.m., you develop feelings about my request. If you hate walking, odds are you are going to tell me that you "want to walk, but just can't squeeze it in." Even if your schedule is wide open, you made your decision because of how you felt about the request.

Our brain and emotions are 90 percent programmed to feel a certain way about most everything before the age of three. For example, if your parents always used food to reward your family when things went well, odds are you instinctively do the same. Every time you accomplished something that pleased them, they gave you a cookie. Now, as an adult, when life is going well, you treat yourself to sweets.

What about when things aren't going so well? Did your parents try to comfort you with food? Maybe every time you were sick, they got you fast-food because it was the only thing you would eat. Now as an adult, whenever life gets rough, for some crazy reason you crave fast-food.

Another common example is always finishing the food on your plate. If you grew up with parents that had to endure the Great Depression, they may have had rules in your home that you had to eat everything on your plate – or else. On the flip side, you may have grown up in a home that didn't always have enough food.

Whatever the reason is, you may just automatically clean your plate whether you are hungry or not. Unintentionally, you may have learned to ignore that little voice inside that tells you when you are hungry, satisfied, and full. After all, you had to learn to ignore it if listening to it got you in trouble.

We all have a history, and that is part of what led us to where we are today. I am here to tell you that this is not your fault. Our learned behaviors explain why we do the things we do. I know that I felt better knowing that I was experiencing normal behaviors – and that I didn't have weak willpower.

The good news is that you can change your programming. You don't have to continue down that old road if it's not where you want to go. We all have the choice to change our course.

Now is the time to accept your past. After all, it has helped you in more ways than you realize; and it has made you who you are. But if there are habits in your past that will not lead you toward your goals, then let's upgrade and replace them with new and improved actions. Give yourself *permission* to leave your baggage at the door of your past. You don't have to haul it around anymore. Your past does not need to determine your future.

In Darkness, Your Light Will Shine

Have you ever been backed into a corner, and you came out swinging? You had no idea you had that much strength! This reminds me of my client, Tony. He was referred to me by his kidney doctor, a colleague of mine. Tony had received an organ transplant 20 years ago. When he got the transplant, he felt so blessed to have a second chance at life.

Tony watched what he ate, and started walking. He was doing great and his transplant doctor was happy. Tony thought that since he was doing so well, he should "treat" himself more often. After all, doesn't he deserve to enjoy life? The problem started when his weekly ice cream trip turned into daily fast-food trips. Before he knew it, he started feeling tired. His joints began hurting, and he used that as an excuse to stop walking. He supposed he didn't feel that bad for just sitting around the house all day.

This went on for a few years and Tony didn't think much of it. It became his new normal. He ate whatever tasted good whenever he wanted. This seemed fine, until one day while visiting the transplant center, Tony was told that he was in danger of losing his transplant. He didn't even realize he had packed on over 40 pounds, and all this extra weight was putting too much stress on his organs. To make matters worse, the doctor told him his blood sugar, blood pressure, and cholesterol were all too high, and he needed to start taking medications to control them.

Tony was scared. How could this happen? He was already taking enough medication, and was desperate for another solution. He asked his doctor what else he could do.

That next week Tony and I started working together. It wasn't until he was backed into that corner that he came out swinging. He was ready to make changes and stick to them. As you can imagine, Tony felt like a failure. Here he had been lucky enough to get a second chance at life, and he had almost lost it. He started to question if he was even worth it. As we talked, it became apparent that Tony had lost hope. Even though he wanted so badly to save his kidney, he thought he would just fail again. "So, what's the point?" he asked.

The initial consultation with Tony continued on, and I collected enough information to develop a plan tailored to his needs. Before I ended the session, I asked him how he thought I could best help him. His answer may surprise you.

"I think what I need most is for someone to believe in me," Tony said.

Haven't we all felt like this before? The first step in changing is believing that there is a chance you will succeed. If you feel like you will fail, then you probably will. Our emotions dictate our actions.

The great news is, you have a choice in how you feel. You have the power to notice how you feel and decide to continue feeling that way, or to change that feeling. I know that this is harder said than done. This is a skill that has to be practiced day in and day out. I have been practicing for years, and still find my emotions sometimes ruin things. We aren't machines. Effecting change takes time.

The first step is being willing to try, and choosing to believe in a positive outcome. Every day. I am here to tell you, that you can change the way you feel, the way you think – and ultimately - the way you live.

Over the next year, Tony decided to grow his belief in himself by setting goals and working toward them. At each session, he was genuinely surprised when he achieved another goal. And then, he started setting – and achieving - more challenging goals. In the darkness of possibly losing his life, his light shined bright. Today, Tony has reached (and maintains) his goal weight. He saved his transplant. He had no idea how strong he was, until he had to be.

Chapter 3
Setting Realistic Goals

The first step in progressing toward a goal, is making a goal. I'm not talking about a generic goal, such as wanting to lose weight and feel better. I am talking about very specific goals: eating five vegetables each day; walking five days each week; and losing 20 pounds by New Year's Day.

Your goals need to be specific, with measureable actions and realistic deadlines. It's normal to want to achieve that perfect weight and feel amazing as soon as possible, but reality is that change takes time. The quick fixes obviously don't work. Anything valuable takes time and effort. So if you truly value this goal, give yourself an appropriate amount of time.

Have you ever watched a toddler when they are just learning to walk? They stand up, and fall down; stand up, and fall down again. They may get brave and try to take a few steps, but fall again. Do we get frustrated with them that they don't go from crawling to walking perfectly over night? Of course not. So why do we get so frustrated with ourselves when we try to learn new things?

It is natural to want results fast, especially in today's immediate gratification environment. Years ago, if you wanted to read a certain book, you may have had to go to the library to check it out. If one library didn't have it, you might have driven to another library, or put your name on a waiting list. A week or two later, the library would call you to say your book is in. When life was moving at a slower pace, we had more patience.

Nowadays, if you want a certain book, Amazon can deliver it to your door the same day; or you can download it immediately to your Kindle. Technology is a wonderful and useful tool; however, it may cause us to lose patience with life – and even ourselves.

A healthy weight loss is around one or two pounds per week – not 40 pounds in 40 days (or whatever the latest commercial is touting). Those programs leave you feeling horrible and irritable. You may lose a little weight, but odds are your energy is cut so low that your metabolism slows down. After you just can't take any more of the program, you go back to your normal routines and gain all that weight back...plus a little more. Sound familiar?

Our bodies are not machines; we have determined that. Instead, they are more like plants, and require a delicate balance of nutrients, water, sunlight, and more. Plants go through different seasons, when they grow more or less, or produce flowers or fruit.

Our human bodies have similar components that go through different seasons due to our emotional, physical, and hormonal needs. That's right, I said hormones. No matter your age, we all have hormones and it is extremely common for those hormones to be thrown off.

Major and minor life events, food, and even exercise can cause those hormones to become out of kilter. To combat this lack of balance, you may need to eat more often, or step up your workouts. These new actions turn to habits, and the weight starts falling off - hallelujah! But then all of a sudden, the weight loss stops (or you may even gain a few pounds). What happened?

You are doing everything the same, so why did your new habits stop working? Hormones probably happened. Maybe you just took on new responsibility at work; or your teenager is stressing you out; perhaps your spouse started golfing and now your schedule has been changed. Things like this can throw your hormones out of balance, which can affect weight loss. Don't worry! By learning to listen to your body through awareness, reflection, and making small adjustments, you can bring things back into symmetry so your progress can continue.

Chapter 4
Understanding Hormones – Balance Them To Burn Fat

Over the years, I have worked with many wonderful people and I have learned as much from them as they have from me. One of the key lessons I have learned, is that we are not machines. Calories in vs. calories out is not the only factor in losing weight.

A great example of this comes from Bonnie, a past client of mine. Bonnie had a Type-A personality, if you know what I mean. She loved the structure of a nutrition plan, but was frustrated that her years of calorie restriction and exercising had not led to the weight loss or energy she was looking for. She was ready to give up. Bonnie told me that her metabolism was "broken," and that she was just going to have to accept this. She was never going to have the body that fit with the calories she ate.

The more Bonnie shared, the more intently I listened. By the end of the conversation, she told me she was surprised that I didn't respond the way her doctors previously had. She expected me to repeat their recommendations – to eat less and workout harder if she wasn't losing weight. Instead, I had her take a hormone assessment questionnaire designed by the incredibly knowledgeable Doctor of Obstetrics, Sara Gottfried, M.D. Just as I suspected, her hormones were out of balance.

After reviewing her results, I explained to her that the stress from work and an over-restricted food intake had caused her cortisol (stress hormone) level to rise too high; and her thyroid (metabolism) level, to plummet too low.

Bonnie was accidentally slowing her metabolism down by reducing her calorie and nutrient intake too much. And that hour of intense cardio at the gym was also raising her cortisol level. This combination was not resulting in weight loss because her physical body thought it was in so much distress, that it was going to starve to death.

When our bodies are stressed and undernourished, they go into defense mode and start storing our food intake. This causes us to maintain or gain weight, instead of letting go of it. When cortisol is elevated, it decreases our metabolic rate. So, it is helpful to increase your intake of cortisol-decreasing foods (like healthy fats); and decrease your intake of cortisol-elevating foods (like processed carbohydrates).

Bonnie sat there staring at me in disbelief. No wonder her body wasn't letting go of the extra pounds, it was trying to protect her against a drought. Bonnie went on to tell me that she felt like she was in starvation mode; she had no energy and was basically miserable.

So I asked Bonnie to try something new. Instead of regulating her intake based on caloric amounts, I recommended little changes like only eating when she was hungry; reducing processed carbohydrates; and doing more resistance training and less cardio.

Bonnie didn't see how making little changes could get the results she wanted, but what she was doing was making her miserable, so she decided to give it a try.

Those crazy, over-restrictive diets haven't worked in the past, and they are not going to work now. I challenge you to choose to drop the baggage of your past at the door - and leave it there.

Let's try something new! What do you have to lose? You have so much more to gain, like self-forgiveness, self-love, and, of course, shedding those extra pounds.

Chapter 5
Don't Let Negative Feelings Run Your Life

What you have read so far may make you think you need to be more self-aware. You may also think that you are totally self-aware, or you wouldn't have bought this book! You are reminded of your "awareness" every time you get dressed, walk past a mirror, or think about eating. And, you are right. We are aware of physical issues because we can see, touch and feel them. But what about the issues that we can't see, touch or feel?

I am talking about our thoughts and feelings. We all have that little voice in our head that tells us mean things. Karey, a recent client of mine, described it very clearly.

"It's like the right half of my brain is telling me how horrible I am, and how disgusting I look. So, why even try to change? I am just going to fail. I am not worth the effort," Karey said.

Let's call that right side of the brain the "negative voice." I asked Karey if the left side of her brain had a voice, too. She sat there for a few minutes and pondered. Then, Karey took a deep breath, and said she used to hear a voice from that side, but not for some time. She went on to say, "It feels like when you have a good friend that you haven't seen in a while."

Karey was very accurate in her description of the thoughts and feelings she was having in her mind. We all have those two voices. One voice puts us down and says we are not good enough. That voice may come from your childhood, friends or family, and especially from society today.

Watch almost any television show, or check out any magazine. The people in them are very often portrayed as unrealistically beautiful, and incredibly thin. Not only do these people have personal trainers, chefs, and therapists to provide all the support they need, but they also have professional photographers who get just the right angles and light (not to mention Photo Shop). How can we expect to look like those societal images, when those people don't even look like those people?

It is normal to have these thoughts. We are surrounded by a society that has unrealistic expectations - which is why that voice can sound so loud and feel so harsh. The great news is, just like Karey, we all have that other, kinder, voice in our minds as well.

If you are like Karey, and haven't heard that voice in a while, listen to the way you speak to the people that you love. I asked Karey who she enjoys spending time with, and she mentioned her grandchildren. She use to have lots of girlfriends she liked to spend time with, but over the years, the negative voice in her head got so loud that she distanced herself from them. Now, the only people she enjoyed were her daughter and grandchildren.

I asked Karey what she likes to do with them. She said she likes to take them to the park and help them play. The grandchildren were young, and needed help climbing on the playground equipment and being pushed on the swings. I asked if they ever fell down and needed help getting up.

"Of course they do; they fall all the time. I just pick them up, wipe them off, and tell them it's okay – just try again," Karey naturally responded.

You may have a friend or family member you support in the same way. Whether they are children or adults, you provide nurturing support when they need it. Pay attention to your voice when you are speaking to that person. Notice the tone, the volume, and the sincerity you communicate with. That voice you are using is the "positive voice" that we all have inside us. That is the voice Karey refers to as her "left brain voice."

In the past, before we were brainwashed by our environment, we had this positive voice inside us that told us to get up when we fell down. It told us to be brave, take those first steps and play with other kids - even if we all looked different and had various capabilities on the playground. The differences didn't slow us down, because we had that inner voice telling us, "It's okay, just keep going."

As adults, we tend to lose communication with that voice. The rest of our world gets so loud that all we can focus on is the negativity. It is extremely important to reconnect with your positive voice. Once you find it, nurture it. It can be very helpful to journal positive thoughts daily.

Karey decided to jot down all of the things she was proud of each day. At first, her journal had entries like, "I am proud of getting out of bed, going to work, and doing the dishes." After a few weeks, she set new goals and her entries changed to, "I am excited that I walked a mile. I can't believe it. If felt so good to be outside."

Over the months, Karey started thinking more positively. She became better at turning down the volume of her negative voice. When it tried to sneak back in, Karey pulled out her journal and read her entries aloud.

"Sometimes I even say them over and over. Sometimes I have to shout out loud that I am happy, and I am proud of myself, in order to hear my positive voice and put my negative voice on mute," said Karey.

I encourage you to do the same. Find that voice. Write about it. Talk about it. Shout about it. Do whatever you have to do to hear it and believe it. Do it daily. This will help you reprogram your brain, and gain the confidence to set new goals and achieve them.

Continue or Change

I challenge you to reconnect with that positive inner voice. If you haven't heard it in a while, put yourself in a situation with others you naturally nurture and support. Practice listening to how you speak to them. Spend more time with them so you can practice more often. At first, it might be like walking through a crowd and seeing a glimpse of your old cherished friend. Memories of good times might come flooding back, or they might just flash by like a dream you vaguely remember having.

Continue this process until you feel like you have a true grasp on that positive voice; and that you can call upon it whenever you need it. It is important to reconnect and practice using this voice with others, because the next step can feel a bit strange.

This important next step is to intentionally start speaking to yourself with that positive voice. If at first you don't know what to say, it can be helpful to write down a list of the top three things your negative voice says to you (those little thoughts that go through your mind often). Now write down the direct opposite of those thoughts.

For example, Karey heard her negative voice saying she was tired, fat, and unworthy. We turned those statements around to say she was energized, healthy, and valuable. Your statements can be anything. Make them your own.

Moving Forward

Now that you have a positive affirmation, write it down and say it to yourself ten times each morning, and ten times each evening. At first, this will probably feel a little phony – and maybe even cheesy – but that is normal. You may feel that way because you haven't yet begun to trust and believe in those statements.

The beauty in the process is that writing and verbalizing these statements daily can help you reprogram the thoughts and emotions that have been ingrained in you so deeply since birth. It's like turning up the volume on the positive voice, and turning down the volume on the negative voice. I wish there was a way to mute the negative voice, but I feel it is there to keep us in check; after all, life is about balance.

This process also increases awareness of our thoughts and feelings. Every time our negative voice rears its ugly head, we can say, write, or even yell our positive affirmations from the roof tops. Practicing this daily will speed up the process. You may even want to check in with your thoughts and feelings a few times a day to see where you are at. If you notice the negative voice is the only one doing the talking, fight back. Actively speak to your positive voice! Awareness of thoughts and choosing to change them is one of the most powerful tools we have.

Imagine yourself achieving your goals. If you really believe that you can, wouldn't it be easier to take the actions you need to get there? After all, now that you are aware of your positive and negative voices, you have the power to continue down that negative road - or take the positive off-ramp toward your goal.

A great way to enter this positive frame of mind, is to close your eyes and imagine yourself after you have already obtained your goal. Think about what you would look like. How would you be different? Would your skin be glowing and bright? Would your hair and nails be strong and shiny? What size would you feel comfortable at?

Now imagine how you feel at that goal. Do you feel strong, healthy and happy? How much energy do you have? What would it feel like to have that energy and strength? How would that help you in your life?

I asked these same questions to my client, Karen, and like her, you may feel a little overwhelmed. She noticed that deep down, she never believed that she could actually accomplish her goals. When I asked her to imagine what it would look like and feel like to achieve her goals, she couldn't picture them. How could she move forward in physical actions, if she didn't really believe in herself?

Instead of discussing what she wanted to change about her food intake, Karen and I spent the whole session developing her thoughts on the possibility of success. These questions are not easy; they are not meant to be. They are meant to help expand our minds and possibly change perspectives from impossible to possible.

I am not saying we are all going to achieve our goals as long as we believe. After all, we might not have healthy or realistic goals in the first place. My point is, that if we don't believe our goals are possible, then we set ourselves up for failure before we even begin. If we believe in ourselves, we can at least make progress and we are encouraged to keep trying. Remaining complacent in our thoughts only leads us to remain complacent in our action.

Now is the time to put in the mental and emotional work so that your actions become purposeful. I have helped thousands of people achieve their goals; why can't the next person be you? Give yourself permission to dream. To imagine. To change perspective for the better. And to find success. It's not always easy, but it is most certainly possible.

Nourish Your Body

Now that we have reconnected with our positive inner voice, it will be easier to move forward with the next step. We are learning how to take better care of ourselves, and that includes not only nourishing our minds, but nourishing our bodies – we are worth it!

The physical human body is just like any other animal on the planet. We all need air to breathe, food to eat, water to drink, nights to sleep, and physical activity to keep us moving. Although we have been blessed with the ability to use our minds to put a man on the moon, physically we are no different than our pets.

Let's begin our focus on food. Why do we eat? That's a great question to ask yourself before each snack or meal. Are you actually feeling hungry? What physical symptoms do you experience when you are hungry?

Common symptoms are a growling stomach, or feeling empty, tired, shaky, or weak. This is because our bodies need energy and we must fuel them. Would you expect your car to take you to work if you didn't put any gas in the tank? Of course not, yet so many of us expect our bodies to keep working without the proper food.

We must learn to actually *nourish* our bodies.

PART II
NOURISH YOUR BODY

Chapter 6
The Metabolism Miracle – Rev It Up!

One of the most common questions I get is, "What is a metabolism, and how can I make it go faster?"

Your metabolism is the rate at which your body converts food to fuel. I often refer to metabolism as calorie burning, interchanging words such as food, fuel, and energy.

Despite what we have been told about losing weight, drastically cutting calories and spending hours at the gym doesn't work. It can actually slow down your metabolism – or calorie burning. At this point, your body will start fighting against you because you are accidentally forcing it into fat-storing mode, delaying weight loss, or even causing weight gain. Yikes! Can you believe it?

It's not that you aren't trying hard enough, or that your metabolism is "broken" from years of dieting. It's just that you need to switch your body from fat-storing mode, to fat-burning mode. In order to go into fat-burning mode and stay there, you actually have to eat more then you're probably eating now. Your body needs to regain trust in you.

When you cut calories too much, or go too long in between meals (even if you're not hungry), your body gets concerned and begins storing fat for a famine. When you think about it, this is ingenious. It's why our ancestors didn't starve to death during times of inadequate food supplies. Think back to those who may have endured the Great Depression; for most, there simply wasn't enough food - and their bodies adapted.

Our body's resourcefulness is amazing, but when you don't feed it properly, that storing mode will get in the way of desired weight loss. The way to outsmart a very smart system is to keep that metabolism burning the right way. It's like taking it from a slow, hybrid engine, to a gas-guzzling V8 Mustang engine.

A classic example of this is my long-term client, Sherry. Sherry had been desperately trying to lose about 20 pounds for the last few years. She believed food was making her fat, so she cut way back on eating. One day she told me how horrible she was feeling with headaches and fatigue. After going through her normal daily food intake, it became very clear that Sherry was feeling so poorly because she had cut her food intake down to about 800 calories or less each day. No wonder she wasn't losing weight; her body was in starvation/survival mode, trying to store everything in an effort to sustain life.

Sherry's headaches were a result of her restricted caloric intake. Her body was breaking down its muscle and fat stores in order to provide carbohydrates to support brain function. This process is called catabolism, and can lead to decreased muscle mass and even organ damage.

Sherry just couldn't understand how she could be eating so little, and still gain weight. She felt like she had tried everything: limiting her food (even though she was hungry), and exercising daily – yet she couldn't lose a single pound. She felt awful physically, and hopeless.

After a few sessions, Sherry agreed that what she had been doing wasn't ever going to work. She agreed to try eating a little more, and to begin listening to her body instead of ignoring it.

Sherry expressed her concern that eating more would cause her to gain even more weight, but said, "What the heck. What I've been doing for years isn't working; what do I have to lose?" Sherry began to listen to what her body had to say, instead of treating it like it was the enemy. She started by adding in more fruits and vegetables, and soon after was adding in more proteins and healthy fats.

To Sherry's surprise, not only was she starting to feel better, but the pounds finally started to fall off. The next time she came to my office to share her results, tears rolled down her face.

"How in the world is this possible," Sherry said. "How am I able to eat more, feel better, and still lose weight? This doesn't make any sense to me."

Sherry was just shocked – but happy. Her headaches were less frequent and her energy was increasing. She didn't even need an afternoon nap anymore. And after a few weeks, Sherry started walking and biking daily. Although she still couldn't wrap her mind around the concept that eating more was helping her, she decided that since it was working, she would go ahead and continue down this road.

As time passed, Sherry noticed that the more she listened to her body, the more balanced she ate, and the better she felt. She went from having chronic migraines where she couldn't even get off the couch for days, to walking, biking, swimming, and doing yoga daily. Sherry now cooks for her family each day, too. They no longer depend on processed food. Replacing chips with nutritious fruit and nuts, and bread with green, leafy lettuce, has helped Sherry and her family gain energy and shed the extra weight.

Now that Sherry and her family are feeling better, they have become more involved in church and have started a youth program. Sherry has literally regained her life with small changes, like balancing her food intake and listening to her body.

Isn't that your objective as well? To not only achieve your health and weight goals, but to have the energy to live the life you want to live.

My goal for all of my clients is to help them regain control of their lives, and increase their energy levels so they can think, feel and be present in life. Enjoy your life!

Chapter 7
Honor Your Hunger; Respect Your Fullness

Don't let life pass you by. We only get one shot, so let's make it count!

Feed your body when it is hungry. Stop when you are just starting to feel full. It takes about 15 minutes for your stomach to send signals to your brain that you are full, so slow down. Break halfway through eating to take a drink, take a few deep breaths, or maybe chat with a friend. By slowing down, not only do you give your body a chance at working correctly, you also get more time to enjoy the delicious food you are eating.

So what are you going to do? You have to make a change, right? Decide right here, and right now, that you are going to stop starving your body.

It's helpful to start by feeding your body small portions every few hours. This may be hard at first if you are not used to it, but the more often you fuel your body in this way, the easier it gets.

This small action will actually speed up your metabolism. Your body will start burning calories at a faster rate. Your energy levels will begin to soar. This system is going to help you shed those extra pounds, and keep them off for the rest of your life. Stop doing fad diets and short-term quick fixes. They don't work. Instead, aim for a lifestyle that will have you feeling amazing. Are you ready?

Chapter 8
Calories: Quality Vs. Quantity

If limiting calories and exercising were the only factors in losing weight, we would all be the perfect size. But there is more to it than just calories. It's about the types of calories we are eating.

Calories can be broken down into three major groups: carbohydrates, proteins, and fats. The best sources of these components are natural, untampered-with sources.

Great carbohydrate choices are organic fruits and vegetables. Although they are becoming more main stream, organics can still be a little pricey. Growing your own garden – big or small – is not only fun, but it can help supplement your groceries (and you know exactly where your produce is coming from!). If you grow more than you can eat, you can always freeze the extras.

The best protein sources are hormone and antibiotic-free, grass-fed animal proteins like eggs and meats. Animal protein is the only protein that can instantly honor the needs of the body. The differences in animal and plant proteins will be discussed in an upcoming chapter.

Last, but not least, are healthy fats like olive oil, avocados, butter, nuts, and seeds. These natural fats are vital in balancing our blood sugar and hormones, so don't leave them out.

In order to feel great and stay in that fat-burning mode, it is important to enjoy all three of these main food groups with each meal.

Chapter 9
Carbohydrates: Think Energy

Carbohydrates give us energy. We actually need these macronutrients to live. Despite what we have been told, carbohydrates are not the enemy. They give us energy by converting into sugar – or fuel – for our bodies.

There are two types of carbs: Fast and Slow. You will find Fast (or "Simple") carbs in foods such as bread, chips, crackers, pasta, sweets, plain old sugar, and other foods that are processed or starchy. Slow (or "Complex") carbs are found in fruits, vegetables, legumes, grains, and dairy products.

Fast carbs turn to sugar quickly, and send our blood sugar skyrocketing (with a crash back down to earth). Imagine a rocket. Eating, say, a big plate of pasta, is like loading our body with rocket fuel, causing our blood sugar to blast off. The problem is, that most of the time we are not fueling for the blast off of a marathon or something similar, but just a simple (non-active) meal. What happens when all that rocket fuel isn't used? Our bodies convert it to fat for storage.

Insulin: Our Fat-storing Hormone

When we eat too many carbs at one time, we go into fat-storing mode. This process begins with the conversion of carbohydrates to sugar for fuel. Our bodies, sensing the rise in sugar, sends out for a hormone called insulin, from our pancreas. Insulin's job is to escort the sugar to our cells.

Picture a large crowd of people waiting to get into a concert. Just like the ushers that direct people to their seats, the insulin ushers the sugar into our cells (without it, the sugar gets stuck in the bloodstream). Our body then assesses if it needs the fuel right at that moment or not. If not, the sugar is stored as body fat. The more carbs we eat, the more insulin we make, the more fat we store. And what goes up, must come down. When that rocket fuel isn't used, it all comes crashing back to earth. You may have noticed that after a big meal by feeling tired, irritable, or just plain needing a nap.

Unfortunately, the more sweets or starchy foods you eat, the more you crave. That's because your blood sugar is rising and falling at a rapid pace. I often refer to this as the blood sugar roller coaster. The more we eat, the higher we go and the harder we fall. Although roller coasters at a theme park are fun, imagine being stuck on one that keeps going and going. How exhausting would that be? No wonder we can become tired and lethargic by the end of the day. Our bodies have spent so much energy trying to control that roller coaster, that there isn't enough vigor left to cook dinner or take that evening walk.

You probably have heard of insulin before. These days it is a more common term, especially since the rise in diabetes has caused an increased need for injectable insulin. It seems like you can't watch television without seeing several medicine commercials in a short period of time.

If we constantly overload our bodies with starch or stress, the insulin created by our pancreas becomes less effective. We actually build up a resistance to it, and our bodies have to work harder to make more insulin.

Remember the "I Love Lucy" episode where Lucy was working at the chocolate factory? At first, she and Ethyl are sitting at the slow-moving conveyer belt placing chocolates in wrappers.

"This is easy! We can handle this," Lucy says. But then the conveyer belt speeds up. The chocolates come out faster and faster, and no matter how desperately they try to keep up, they can't.

This is what happens when we overload our body with carbohydrates and sugar. Our pancreas starts making poor quality insulin, and our bodies are unable to use it. So what happens to all that sugar? It gets stuck floating around in our bloodstream. You might be thinking, so what? Unfortunately, that excess sugar acts more like battery acid. It starts eating away at our blood vessels, nerves, and organs. The excess can also lead to high blood sugar, or Diabetes.

When blood sugar is high for an extended period of time, not only do we gain weight, but permanent damage is being caused to our bodies. Common symptoms of high blood sugar levels are feeling tired, thirsty, hungry, having blurred vision, and more. The scary thing is, many of us are walking around with this condition and either aren't paying attention to the symptoms, or don't have any symptoms at all. Despite feeling fine, the sugar may be causing irreversible blindness, kidney failure, heart disease, cancer, and more. Diabetes is known as a silent killer for good reason!

If you would like to get out the fat-storing mode and into the fat-burning mode, then it is necessary to cut down on these carbohydrates, and increase our protein and fat intake. The first step is to eliminate processed foods such as breads, candies, cereals, chips, cookies, pastas, pastries, and pretzels. I know, they are quick and yummy – but they trigger more fat storage.

If it is not something that you can pick from a garden or pull off a tree, then odds are it's processed. The problem with these foods is that they are two to three times higher in carbs than natural foods. They send our blood sugar soaring, only to crash and crave more of them. It's all too easy to get stuck in this viscous cycle, leaving us feeling tired and miserable. Nobody wants to live this way.

If you want a clear mind, energized body, and enjoy sound sleep – cut out the processed foods!

Portion Control

Since the right carbohydrates give us energy, they are important to enjoy with each meal and snack. Limit your portions to one-half to one cup per serving, with the exception of non-starchy vegetables.

Non-starchy vegetables include everything other than beans, corn, peas, potatoes, sweet potatoes, plantains, and squash. These particular vegetables listed are higher in carbs, and do spike blood sugar and insulin levels. Enjoy them in moderation. Non-starchy vegetables – like leafy greens - are high in antioxidants and fiber, and help us feel full. Fill up at least half your plate with them and enjoy!

Enjoy: Fruits; vegetables.

Limit: Starchy vegetables (listed above); whole grains (barley, beans, brown rice, bulger, legumes, lentils, oats, quinoa); dairy (milk, yogurt).

Avoid: High Fructose Corn Syrup, sugars, agave nectars; all processed foods.

For a complete grocery list and nutritional coaching, contact us at www.thrivenutritionandfitness.com.

Chapter 10
Proteins: The Building Blocks of Life

The next macronutrient our bodies need is protein. Proteins are the building blocks of life. We need them to build and repair tissues, make healthy new cells, hormones, and enzymes. And they are very important to our organs, bones, blood, skin, and nails.

Proteins are also high in vitamin B, which gives us energy and strength. They not only feed our muscles, they feed our brains, too. The brain uses proteins that we consume to communicate its needs between the neurons.

Imagine the proteins as our emails. You can write an email, but if you don't have a way to send it, then it's useless. Proteins act as our email provider, taking our messages and delivering them to the recipients.

If you are not eating enough protein, your thinking may be foggy, your body may feel tired, and your muscles will disappear. If you are having cravings for things like chocolate or nuts, odds are you may have a magnesium deficiency – also known as eating too many carbohydrates and not enough proteins. Boost your protein intake to curb those cravings.

Proteins can be broken up into two categories: plant proteins and animal proteins. The most common plant proteins are beans, lentils, legumes, soy, and whole grains. Since nuts and seeds are higher in fat, they get placed in the healthy fat category.

The problem with plant-based proteins is that they are not complete proteins. Imagine constructing a puzzle. Each plant protein puzzle has a few pieces that are left out, leaving it unfinished. We need an additional nine essential amino acids - to pair them with the 11 amino acids that our bodies already produce – to construct the complete protein puzzle. Plant proteins, such as beans and grains, are also higher in carbohydrates, and you would need to consume excess amounts just to get an adequate amount of protein.

Soy, another common plant protein, is not only high in carbs, but it can increase your estrogen levels, throwing off vital hormone balances and slowing down your metabolism.

If you prefer not to consume animal protein, you will need to pair grains and legumes so your body can get the right balance of protein. Grains, like rice, corn, bran, wheat, and barley do not contain enough of the essential amino acid, lysine. Legumes, like beans, peanuts, peas, and lentils do not contain enough tryptophan, methionine, or cysteine. The problem is, in order to get enough protein from these sources, you would need to eat four times the recommended amount of carbohydrates per meal.

If you still prefer not to consume animal proteins, you will need to supplement vitamin B12 and magnesium.

Animal proteins contain all 20 amino acids, and are ready for the body to use as needed as soon as they are digested. They also do not contain any carbohydrates, and will help keep you off the blood sugar roller coaster.

Examples of animal proteins are grass-fed, hormone and antibiotic-free meats, chicken and turkey; wild-caught fish; and organic, hormone-free eggs and dairy.

Animal proteins can quickly start rebuilding and repairing damaged cells and muscles, and are shown to boost metabolism higher and longer than plant proteins. If you are looking to boost your calorie burning, animal proteins can help. They are also used by the neurotransmitters in our brains to transfer information so we can think clearly.

It is important to consume enough protein to repair and rebuild our bodies. The wear and tear we put upon ourselves leads to breakdowns, which are often manifested by feeling tired, lethargic, irritable, or even achy. This is our body's way of waving a red flag ("Hello? I need a little help here!").

Another reason for consuming the proper amounts of complete proteins is that our organs are made of protein. Being out of balance forces the body to break down muscles to sustain organ function. After the muscle stores are depleted, the body will start to break down the lesser organs to keep the most vital ones alive. Yikes! This catabolism is something we want to stay far away from.

In order to ensure you are consuming adequate protein, the recommended serving size is four to six ounces (about the size of your palm) of animal protein per meal; and one to two ounces (about the size of one or two of your thumbs) per snack. If you are looking to build muscle, you may require a little more, but make sure you are lifting weights to justify it. Lifting weights tells your body to use that protein to repair and build muscle – otherwise, that extra protein is converted to fat for storage.

Also be sure not to exceed ten ounces of protein per serving, as the body becomes overwhelmed by the excess. It will break down the protein molecules and convert them to sugar to protect itself. Excess protein is processed through the kidneys, so too much can lead to permanent kidney damage. A common sign of excess protein intake is foamy urine. So if you notice this side effect, cut back on the protein.

Protein Supplements

Some people shy away from supplements, hoping to get all their nutritional needs from whole foods. That is a great thought, and I wish it was that easy. But the truth is, consuming adequate amounts of vitamins, minerals, and proteins can be difficult. You would need to consume a wide variety of food, and it takes a lot of time to prepare the proper meals and snacks – not to mention how depleted our resources are. Our topsoil has only a fraction of the minerals that it used to, resulting in a growing environment devoid of nutrients.

Most of us have elevated blood sugar in the morning. It's our body's way of giving us the energy we need to get ready and moving. Having a high protein/low carb breakfast will help you feel full for a longer period of time, and give you the lasting energy needed throughout your day.

I recommend using protein meal shakes. Personally, I drink a shake every morning. It can be so crazy trying to get my family ready and myself off to work, that I often don't have time to make the high protein my body needs.

Choosing a protein supplement can be a little tricky. Most of the supplements sold at our local stores include chemically poisonous fillers, additives, preservatives, and artificial sweeteners. All of these ingredients will increase inflammation in your body and slow down your weight loss - and can even cause weight gain!

Most of these protein supplements also contain denatured protein. This means the whey has been heated to incredibly high temperatures, which breaks down the protein structure and decreases its value to our body.

I recommend pure, clean protein supplements that are free of these harmful ingredients and contain undenatured protein sourced from New Zealand. New Zealand has the strictest dairy standards, and their cows are hormone and antibiotic free. They roam in fields of grass, and produce the purest milk in the world.

When you are extracting and condensing ingredients like whey protein, it is incredibly important to confirm that the ingredients start out pure. Utilizing sub-quality, hormone-filled milk will result in harmful hormone-filled protein powders. Yuck! No one wants that. Another concern is that protein supplements are not regulated by the Food and Drug Administration, so if they are not tested by an independent third party, chances are that the ingredients on the label may not be what is actually in the product.

A recent study of common protein supplements found in our local stores, showed that most of them do not contain the amount of protein stated on the label. If the label showed 25 grams of protein, most actually contained anywhere from six to 20 grams of protein. So what else was in them? Carbs.

If you are going to spend money on a protein supplement, I recommend choosing one that contains pure, undenatured protein; free of chemically made fillers, additives and artificial sweeteners. I use and recommend Isagenix products. They are made with clean, pure, natural ingredients and undenatured protein.

To order these clean and healthy supplements, contact us at www.ThriveNutritionandFitness.com.

Enjoy: Organic, grass-fed, hormone and antibiotic-free meats; wild-caught fish; organic, hormone-free eggs and dairy; and protein meal shakes (supplements).

Avoid: Soy-based products.

Chapter 11
Fat: Bring Back The Flavor!

The third macronutrient we require is fat. That's right, we actually need fat in order for our bodies to function correctly. Back in the 1970s, people decided to start cutting fat out of their diets. It does contain more than twice the calories of other foods, so it's understandable that society thought this would help people lose weight. But as we have learned over the years, eating too many carbohydrates and proteins is not good for us either.

It's no coincidence that ever since we started cutting fat out of our diets, obesity rates have drastically increased. We carry around more weight today than ever before. Too bad we had to learn the hard way that it's not just about the total calories consumed, but more about the quality and type of foods that we are eating.

For years, fat got a bad reputation. You may have felt like it was a forbidden food. "It tastes so good, but watch out!" "Eating fat will make you fat." "A minute on the lips – a lifetime on the hips." These are things we were told over and over again.

Over the years, food companies jumped onto this bandwagon and started manufacturing low-fat and non-fat foods, appealing to this new – albeit incorrect – way of thinking. But in the process of taking out the fat, they took out the flavor as well. In order to make these processed foods taste good, they added in lots of sugar and salt (and some other not so nice things as fillers).

High-fat food sends signals to our brains that we are satisfied and can stop eating. Without fat, we tend to eat more than double normal portion sizes. Have you ever eaten low-fat ice cream? You may have noticed it has much fewer calories - so it's okay if we eat twice as much, right? How did that pan out for us? Since it is lower in fat, we don't feel satisfied as quickly and we tend to eat more...and more...and maybe even some more. And then, we are right back on that blood sugar roller coaster, turning that high-carbohydrate ice cream into fat stores for later.

Despite the reality of the situation, most people are still holding onto their fat-free salad dressings and snacks. A great example of this is my client, George. I have known George for years, and despite his efforts to shed some extra weight, he didn't have much success.

During our first session together, George shared with me how he switched from potato chips to rice cake chips, from regular mayonnaise to non-fat mayo, and from regular cream cheese to non-fat – without losing any weight. With frustration and disappointment in his voice, George quietly said, "How can this be? I have cut hundreds of calories from my intake, but I am still not able to get rid of this belly - and now I feel worse."

George went on to share that his parents were overweight, so it just must be in his genes. He also mentioned an increase in cravings, which led him to eat more of his fat-free options. He rationalized with himself that it wasn't that bad to eat the whole bag of rice cake chips, "Since they were half the calories of potato chips."

After chatting with George for a bit, I shared with him the benefits of healthy fats, and why our bodies need them. They slow down digestion, helping us feel satisfied longer – one of the key reasons George wasn't finding satiety in his non-fat foods. They also help balance our hormones - like the pony express taking important messages from the nervous system throughout the body.

Our bodies use fat for a variety of functions: to coat and protect our cells, brain, hair, skin, and nails. It is essential for every cell in our body, and provides immune support. We need to consume healthy fats in order to absorb fat-soluble vitamins like A, D, E, and K. Without the proper amounts of these vitamins in our system, we can be left feeling tired and sad, and become more susceptible to illness - even cancer.

Fat is vital for our hormone function. Inadequate dietary fat consumption leads to an increase in carbohydrate intake. Taking that ride on the blood sugar roller coaster leads to cravings, irritability, systemic inflammation, and disease. Don't get me wrong, we shouldn't eat unlimited amounts of fat, but a little of the right kind is healthy and necessary.

The healthiest sources of fat are avocados, nuts, olives and olive oils, and seeds. These plant fats are all unsaturated, and high in heart-healthy Omega-3s. Next up, is coconut oil, coconut milk, butter, and cheese - which are saturated fats. There has been a lot of controversy about saturated fats over the years. We use to think they were the cause of blockages in the heart and arteries. Recent research suggests that systemic inflammation is causing the vascular pathways to swell and become blocked.

The key components to reducing systemic inflammation are to reduce your carbohydrate intake, and reduce your stress. Foods high in Omega-3s - like flax and chia seeds, salmon, sardines, and walnuts - all help lower the inflammation that is already there. Try sprinkling a tablespoon of ground flax seeds on your salad or yogurt, or in your protein shake. It doesn't taste like much, but will go straight to work repairing cells and decreasing that systemic inflammation.

The Cholesterol Myth

For years we have been told that cholesterol is bad; that it causes heart attacks and strokes. As a dietitian, I was trained that if a food is hard at room temperature - like butter - then it becomes hard in our bodies. Seems like a reasonable theory, right? Reasonable, until you heat these fats to our normal body temperature of 98.6 degrees, at which point they melt. So, they can't actually harden in our system when our bodies melt them. This simple theory is actually a revolutionary insight for the nutrition world.

The reason we find cholesterol in our arteries is because fat is trying to heal any inflammation it finds. Our hearts and brains are critical for survival, so if inflammation is found in those areas, then the body sends cholesterol to try and heal the location. Think of cholesterol like an ambulance. It rushes around the body tending to the sick areas in an effort to repair the damage and ensure survival. The problem occurs when these areas are inflamed and damaged for long periods of time; they swell up, causing a narrowing in the openings of the arteries. The body sends the cholesterol to try and fix it, but years of accumulation can lead to blockages.

The truth is, heart disease is like many other diseases. It is exacerbated by systemic inflammation made worse by high-carbohydrate, low-fat diets.

Eating Fat Can Help You Slim Down

After sharing this information with George, I asked him how he thought his non-fat foods compared with how he was feeling before. He was stumped. After a few minutes of silence, he let out a big sigh.

"I think I eat more now, and don't feel as well. I just thought it was all in my head. I was trying to cut down my calories and figured that feeling this way was just part of the game; like this was my body's way of punishing me for my poor food choices in the past. I never thought that my current choices could be causing it," George said.

George and I discussed how he could incorporate more healthy fats in his daily intake, and I asked him to track how he felt. Instinctively, George decided to continue tracking his calorie intake along with how his body was feeling. Over the next few weeks, he was blown away. Headaches and irritability had vanished. He noticed he was feeling full more quickly, which caused him to eat less. And, George finally started shedding the belly-fat that was getting in the way of playing with his grandkids.

At our next phone session, George shared that he had been tracking his calories all along. He couldn't believe that he was losing weight, even though he was eating the same amount of calories as before. By just exchanging some starchy carbohydrate foods for healthy fats, he was able to decrease inflammation. His body was able to get to work shedding pounds instead of wasting all that energy repairing the damage and inflammation that was occurring before.

George was experiencing the joy of healthy fats. His brain was getting the signal that he was full and satisfied much sooner than when he was eating all those processed, non-fat carbohydrates. Carbs do not send that signal to the brain until the stomach has reached maximum capacity, so we often end up eating more, but feeling less satisfied.

But before we get carried away, remember that not all fat is good or healthy. Man-made fats are created by heating foods to an extreme temperature to extract the oils. This process causes the fat to partially breakdown and increases its exposure to oxygen. Oxygen and fat do not get along. When fat is exposed to oxygen – or becomes oxidized – it turns harmful. Oxidized fat in cells increases inflammation and the risk of developing cancerous cells. Common oxidized fats are canola, corn, peanut, vegetable and soybean oils. Other fats to avoid are hydrogenated, partially hydrogenated, and trans fats. These are found in fast foods, fried foods, processed snack foods, baked goods, shortening, and margarine.

Portions

The fact that we need the right kinds of fats to be healthy may be an eye-opener to some. It is also important to eat the right portion sizes, as is true with all the foods we eat.

A healthy portion of fat is one to two tablespoons per meal, and one tablespoon per snack. An easy way to visually remember that (without carrying around measuring spoons) is to use your thumbs. The average thumb is about a tablespoon.

So enjoy those avocados, nuts and nut butters, flax seeds and oils, and olives and olive oils – just keep your "measuring spoons" handy. George ended our last session by saying, "I give healthy fats two thumbs up!"

After a year, George reached his goal weight. He also lowered his blood pressure, cholesterol level, and blood sugar. Now, he enjoys apples and nut butter as his daily bedtime snack.

Enjoy: Avocados; organic, grass-fed butter; nuts and nut butters; olives and olive oils; and seeds.

Avoid: Canola, corn, soybean and vegetable oils; hydrogenated and trans fats; margarines; and shortening.

Try pairing a half cup of fruit with one to two tablespoons of cheese, nuts or seeds. Or, sprinkle walnuts in your yogurt, or drizzle olive oil on some sliced tomatoes.

For a complete grocery list and nutritional coaching, contact us at www.thrivenutritionandfitness.com.

Chapter 12
Putting It All Together

Our bodies work best when they get a balance of the three types of fuel they need. Doesn't your car work best when it has quality gas, oil, and other fluids? Asking our bodies to function with inadequate or sub-quality food is like expecting our car to function without oil. I'm not a mechanic, but I'm pretty sure the engine would burn out if we tried to drive our car without oil.

Our bodies are the same. They will burn out if we do not provide them with the food/fuel they need. After all, you probably picked up this book because you feel like you are running on empty and ready to burn out.

Now that we know the portions of the three main nutrients we need, let's build a balanced meal. We should aim to have all three VIP players - carbohydrates, protein, and fat - at each meal. If you visualize your plate, imagine drawing a line right down the middle. Reserve half your plate for non-starchy vegetables. This could include asparagus, broccoli, carrots, zucchini, or salad (the list of delicious veggies is voluminous). Vegetables are high in fiber, vitamins, and minerals. They really are the superhero of the carbohydrate world. Even non-starchy vegetables turn to sugar, but remember that we need carbohydrates (of the right kind) for energy; so eat up!

It can be helpful to start each meal by eating your vegetables first. They require more chewing than starchy foods, like rice, so they start sending signals to the brain that we are eating. The stomach and brain then tell the body to release some insulin, to bring our blood sugars to a healthy energized range.

Feel free to cook your vegetables in one to two tablespoons of extra virgin olive or coconut oil, or top them with a tiny bit of butter and parmesan cheese. These healthy fats will send more signals to the brain so you feel full, faster.

So now we are left with half a plate to fill. Try splitting the remaining space in half again, leaving you with two quarters. One of these quarters is for your protein, and the other is for your carbohydrate. Enjoy a portion of protein about the size of the palm of your hand; and a one-half to one cup portion of carbohydrate (this could be a four to six ounce piece of grilled salmon, with a half cup of red potatoes).

Variety is the spice of life, so mix it up. Opt for two or so servings of wild-caught fish weekly, and fill in the other meals with chicken, beef or turkey. Choose variety with your carbs, too. Ever try using sweet potatoes instead of regular russets? Mash them with some butter and fresh rosemary for a treat. You can even put your whole meal in one bowl. Serve a taco salad with grilled chicken, lots of veggies, a little cheese, and some quinoa – and make a dressing out of salsa, sour cream and some Mexican spices. Delicious!

If you have the opportunity to visit a local farmer's market, you can get fresh, organic fruits and vegetables in season, and build your meal around them. In the summer, my family often skips the starch and we eat more salads because it is so hot in Southern California. I often add berries, apples, corn or beans; and I love a delicious vinaigrette.

Now that we know how to build a balanced meal, we are all good to go, right? Not so fast. It's great that we are learning new things, but there is a little bit more to the story...

As we cut down on starchy carbohydrates, our blood sugars don't go as high, but that means that we need to fuel ourselves more often. Snacks are the secret to success. That's right. I said it. Many of my clients born in the 50s and 60s have been told their whole life that snacks will make you fat. Even when their bodies were screaming, "Feed me!" they were brainwashed to ignore those impulses and wait for the next meal. The problem with this is we arrive starving at our next meal, overeat, and - you guessed it – gain weight.

I am here to tell you, if this is how you were raised, it's not your fault. Ignoring hunger may have been a survival tactic of your parents, especially if they endured the Great Depression of the 1930s. Back then, food was scarce. People had to eat sparingly because there often wasn't enough to go around.

In today's society, we need a new reality. I'll tell you why snacking is a good thing.

Chapter 13
Snacks: The Secret to Success

Compared to the past, the way we currently view food is very different than it was for our parents and grandparents. Today, food is in our faces all day long. It's all over the Internet, social media, television, bill boards...pretty much everywhere. This can make it really hard to resist temptation (and makes us feel guilty if we give in).

The reality is that going too long without eating actually slows down our calorie burning capacity. Skipping snacks - or even meals - can cause us to pack on the pounds. After years of doing this, your body becomes conditioned, and may not even feel hunger anymore.

Many of my clients have often skipped snacks or meals, because they are either too busy, or they thought it would help them lose more weight. All they have done is slow their metabolism down to a crawl. The more time that passes in that state, the longer it takes to get that metabolism up and going again.

Many clients in their 50s and 60s have skipped breakfast and snacks for the past 40 years in an effort to lose weight. It typically takes them six to eight weeks before their bodies regain trust in the food intake, and start burning more calories and shedding pounds. If this is you, don't give up after a week. It took time to get where you are, and it will take time to change things to achieve your goals.

More important than watching the scale, is learning how to listen and care for your body. Eating at least every four hours will rev up your metabolism, causing you to feel a stronger hunger signal. When you hear that signal, don't ignore it! Be prepared with snack options.

Great snack choices are organic fruit, like apples, berries, peaches and pears. These fruit portions should be limited to one-half to one cup servings (about the size of a tennis ball, or less). Pair that fruit with one to two tablespoons of nuts, nut butter, or cheese. These choices are great because you can slip them in a purse or lunch bag; they don't need to be refrigerated and are easy and convenient to eat.

If you have access to a refrigerator (or pack a frozen water bottle in your lunch bag) yogurt or cottage cheese are great choices, too. Just keep the portions at one-half to one cup. I love topping fruit flavored Greek yogurt with one tablespoon of chopped nuts, for a great crunch.

It is best to eat about every three to four hours. If your breakfast is more than four hours from lunch, enjoy a snack between. I find the afternoon and before bed snacks very important. Dinner is often four to six hours after lunch, leaving us with the three o'clock munchies. Be ready with a great snack.

Feeling tired? Pack some protein into your snack, like organic grass-fed jerky or leftover chicken from dinner. The B vitamins will boost your energy and carry you through to dinner. In that regard, limit your protein before bed. Stick with one-half cup of fruit and one tablespoon of fat. I like pear slices and a nice aged cheese.

Snacking not only revs up your metabolism, but it balances those blood sugars while sleeping. Without snacks, we are starving by the time our next meal rolls around, and we gobble up our food way too fast. Snacking keeps us stable and in control, so by the next meal we are hungry, but not starving. We can actually slow down and enjoy our meal, which prevents us from overeating and making poor food choices. After all, when our blood sugar is crashing, human instinct is grab the fastest, easiest thing possible. That's why the fast food industry is booming.

Building a balanced meal is as easy as making sure you have veggies, protein, and healthy fat. The extra half-cup of carbohydrate (or starch) is optional, depending on how you feel. Some days you want it more than others. Somedays you may just want a big salad, or large bowl of chicken and vegetable soup.

The most important thing is to listen to your body. It takes time to adjust, but the more you stick with it, the more quickly you will feel better and achieve your goals. Everyone is different. Some people feel better and progress faster with more protein and less carbohydrates. Some people feel drained of energy and have stalled progress with that, but notice improvement by increasing their healthy carbohydrate portions from one-half to one cup.

These are guidelines that have helped thousands of my clients in the past. One thing I have learned, is that everyone is unique, and requires some adjusting along the way.

Chapter 14
Timing Makes All the Difference

Now that you know how to build a balanced meal, let's chat about timing. You have probably heard that breakfast is the most important meal of the day. Well, I am here to tell you, it really is. I cannot stress this enough. Breakfast is the very thing that boosts your metabolism each day. So if you want to shed some pounds or feel happy and energized, eat something for breakfast.

Our bodies are so well designed that they instinctively know that we are not going to feed them while we are sleeping. And during this seven to nine hours (recommended "Z" time) of critical rest, the body compensates for the lack of fuel by slowing down the rate at which it burns calories – by about 50 percent, actually – and tends to other maintenance. When we awaken the next morning, we are still burning calories at that snail's pace until we eat something. Eye-opening, right? As soon as we feed our bodies, that calorie burning gets turned back up, setting our metabolism into motion.

If you normally skip breakfast, I urge you to get into the habit of eating soon after rising each day, even if it is just a little something. This may feel strange at first, but stick with it even if you are not hungry. If you have busy mornings, you may have trained your body to ignore hunger signals. I have heard every reason in the book, and I believe you. But those who eat within one hour of getting out of bed, always reach a healthy weight faster.

If you are not a "breakfast person," don't worry. I am not recommending you start each day with a 3-egg omelet and a side of pancakes. Something as simple as Greek yogurt with almonds; toast and eggs; or a protein shake will do the trick. It can even be left-overs from last night's dinner. You want to aim for some protein, a half cup of a natural carbohydrate, and one to two tablespoons of a healthy fat. Consuming a healthy balance of food will give you energy, stamina, and focus. Who doesn't need a little more of that each day?

Although balanced meals help us feel great and boost calorie burning, one meal does not last all day. If it does, odds are you over-ate.

Doris came to me a few years ago. She was so frustrated and desperate to lose weight, she cut out breakfast and dinner (she said she wasn't hungry in the morning anyway). After years of working as a nurse - and not having time to eat before or during her job - Doris had become well-trained in ignoring her hunger pangs.

Even 30 years later, Doris just naturally didn't eat in the morning. Her body gave in to the fact that she wasn't going to feed it early on in the day, so it kept her metabolism nice and slow in order to prevent low blood sugar, and perhaps passing out. Doris said that by the time lunch came around, she was pretty hungry, and made that her main meal of the day.

"I figure since it's my only meal of the day, I can eat whatever and however much I want," said Doris at the time. "I usually have a dozen fried chicken wings, coleslaw, and a biscuit with butter and honey. And I can't stand water, so I treat myself to sweet tea."

Doris went on to share that she was rarely hungry for dinner, and since she wanted to lose weight, she skipped that, too. Poor

Doris! So desperate to lose weight that she was willing to cut out meals and snacks. We discussed how eating breakfast works to kick start the daily calorie burning, and it's no surprise that she was floored.

"You mean eating in the morning will help me lose weight? I thought it would make me gain weight!" Doris said.

This is a classic example of one of the misnomers that we have been taught for generations. We now know that skipping meals can help us actually *gain weight.* Breakfast is the best thing to jump start that metabolism – but it doesn't last all day. It is vital to eat every three to four hours during our waking hours to keep our metabolism revved up. This starts from the moment we get out of bed, until we return to it at the end of each day.

A normal day might include three balanced meals with protein, lots of non-starchy vegetables, one-half cup of natural carbohydrates, and one to two tablespoons of a healthy fat at each meal; and two to three snacks in between.

If you feel hunger signals like a growling stomach, dizziness, shakiness, headache or fatigue between meals...then, EAT! This is your body's way of telling you it needs more fuel. When there is not enough fuel, the engine slows down. As a (not so happy) bonus, the fuel goes into fat reserves the next time we eat, just to prevent future starvation.

My typical day usually begins with a protein shake around 6:30 a.m. (I use IsaLean shakes by Isagenix). Protein shakes are great for my busy mornings, when I'm trying to get ready for work and get my children ready for school.

Around 9:00 a.m. (give or take), I'm usually hungry again. My typical snack is apple slices and a small handful of nuts. Lunch is usually around 11:30 a.m., and I always aim to have a balanced meal. I often eat leftovers from the night before, or sliced protein over a large salad.

To prevent that all-too-real afternoon slump, I have another snack at about 2:30 p.m. I vary between hard-boiled eggs, canned tuna, or turkey jerky with a cup of veggies and a little hummus.

My kids are normally starving by 5:00 p.m., so I try to get dinner on the table as soon as possible. Anyone with hungry kids understands, you have to feed them or they can turn wild on you. Children are amazing at listening to their hunger signals. They don't have all the other stress of life weighing them down. And, they don't ignore their hunger – they make it a top priority. This is a great lesson for all of us.

I shared my typical day with Doris, and she laughed at me saying, "How can you eat that much and not gain weight?" I hadn't even mentioned my evening snack to her yet. The truth is, if we feed our bodies, they burn more calories. If we starve our bodies, they burn less calories and store more fat.

Timing is a very important part to helping you feel strong and energized – and timing can help you lose weight. It doesn't matter if you get out of bed at 5 or 10 a.m., try to eat within an hour of waking to boost that calorie burning capacity. Enjoy a balanced meal or snack, including a bit of fruit and vegetables, and a serving of healthy fat. Then eat every three to four hours, as needed. Listen to your body. Somedays you may need more, some days you'll need less.

I asked Doris how she typically felt after lunch, and the answer I got was not surprising: Full, tired and in need of a nap. I also asked her on a sale of 1 to 10 (with ten being stuffed), how she felt after her main meal.

"Since I am normally pretty hungry by lunch, and I know I am going to skip dinner, I guess I eat until I am a ten – totally stuffed to the max," said Doris.

I told Doris that our stomachs are similar to a balloon; they can get stretched out. The more we fill them, the bigger they get (and the more it takes to fill them). When we overeat, our bodies have to spend all their energy digesting that enormous amount of food, trying urgently to lower our excessively high blood sugar. This doesn't leave us with energy to do much else (that food coma feeling you may have experienced after overeating).

It's best to eat when you are just starting to get hungry, at a hunger scale of around three or four. You should stop eating when you are just starting to get full, at around a six. Eating small portions every few hours will drive up that metabolism, give you energy, and keep you in fat-burning mode.

I knew asking Doris to eat three meals and a few snacks each day was way too far from her current state. So I asked her what stood out the most from everything we had discussed.

Doris said, "Now I understand why I'm not eating that much, but still gaining all this weight. I slowed down my metabolism. I think I will start with trying to at least eat three meals a day, and then I will try and work in the snacks later."

Definitely a step in the right direction!

Chapter 15
Stubborn Sticky Pounds and Thyroid Imbalance

How are you doing so far? Have you started trying these changes? If not, there is no better time to start than right now. Don't think about it, just do it. It's too easy to overthink the task and talk yourself right out of it. I bet you can name at least three reasons why you should start at a later date. My question to you is, how many times have you already decided to wait until that perfect moment to start (Monday, next week, the first of the month, the New Year)?

Starting right now is the best thing you can do for yourself. We are all busy, and there will always be a reason to put off your plans. Continuing to carry around this extra weight will lead to permanent damage and disease, so stop planning and start doing.

Alright, maybe you have started making changes; or maybe you are like my client, Stacey. Stacey felt like she was doing everything right. She was monitoring her portions, eating when physically hungry, and drinking more water. Despite her efforts, she couldn't lose a single pound - and was even *gaining* weight.

During her first session with me, Stacey shared, "I am so frustrated. I am trying so hard, but nothing is working. I guess I'm going to have to come to terms with the fact that I am just going to be fat. I feel so defeated. I even went to my doctor and had my thyroid checked, but it came back normal."

This might surprise you, or it might not. Maybe you know exactly how Stacey feels. The good news is, there is hope.

Over the years, I have helped hundreds of clients that had their thyroid checked by their General Practitioner, only to be told that it was WNL (Within Normal Limits). The most common thyroid blood lab test is called the TSH Level - or Thyroid-Stimulating Hormone Level - and it is not a very accurate test. In fact, most clients report many symptoms of an underactive thyroid, even though their levels may show within normal limits. One problem with this particular lab test, is that "normal" covers a broad spectrum. It is quite possible to have normal test results, and still be suffering from an underactive thyroid.

Common symptoms are hair loss; dry or brittle hair, skin and nails; problems losing weight; constipation; feeling cold all the time; chronic fatigue; depression; moodiness; goiter; and a family history of thyroid problems - to name a few.

Stacey reported having most of these problems for the past year. She also went on to share that she had been putting on weight ever since she started feeling this way.

Stacey and I continued by assessing what she ate, her activity level, how much sleep she was getting, her hormone symptoms, and such. By the end of our session, I felt that she was suffering from an underactive thyroid.

An underactive thyroid is becoming more common in my practice. This can feel incredibly frustrating, but the good news is there is something you can do to help balance your thyroid naturally.

The first thing I recommend is cutting out gluten. Gluten is a protein naturally contained in wheat products like bread, crackers, cereal, oatmeal, and even ketchup.

It's helpful to replace those gluten-type carbs with fruits and vegetables. You can also switch to corn chips, corn tortillas, and gluten-free products. Just be careful; gluten-free bread is still bread (empty carbs), so limit the intake.

In general, I recommend limiting or avoiding gluten altogether, since bread and crackers do not contain necessary nutrients. Instead, they are more akin to empty calories that can pack on the pounds.

Some people are more gluten-sensitive, with common symptoms like bloating, constipation, nausea, and weight gain. Gluten is also a protein that can confuse our bodies. In some, it can be interpreted by the body as a foreign substance that instigates a fight. The body will send in little soldiers (antibodies) to go to war with the gluten in the gut. The problem is, when our body is at war, all of our resources and energy are dedicated to winning that battle. This leaves scant energy and resources to repair cells or burn fat.

In short, your body may think of gluten as a terrorist, and as such, waste important resources trying to fight it off. Since gluten is not an essential nutrient, reducing it as much as possible will most likely reduce bloating, increase energy, and stimulate weight loss.

The next nutrient might surprise you, as it is hidden in a lot of products. I'm taking about fluoride. Recent studies are showing an association between increased fluoride exposure and underactive thyroid function. Fluoride is commonly found in toothpaste, mouthwash and tap water.

If we are exposed to too much fluoride, it is likely that we can develop an iodine and selenium deficiency. In order for our thyroids and metabolisms to work efficiently, we need adequate iodine and selenium in our systems.

Too much fluoride can prevent the absorption of iodine and selenium, thus slowing down thyroids and metabolisms. Most of us do not consume enough iodine these days, since many have cut out iodized table salt and switched to sea salt (or avoid salt completely). I recommend switching back to iodized table salt, and enjoying two to four Brazil nuts per day to help increase iodine and selenium levels. Iodine is also found in seaweed, eggs, and dairy products.

If you have tried everything to lose weight, but nothing is working, cut gluten out of your diet, switch to filtered water, and use fluoride-free toothpaste and mouthwash. It can also be helpful to install a water filtration system in your home that specifically removes fluoride, and other contaminants. You can purchase them online or at your local hardware store. We installed one and it dropped the contaminant level from 230 milligrams per liter to 17! What a big difference. The water tastes delicious, and we are saving money by not having to buy bottled water.

Just as gluten and fluoride can wreak havoc on your system, there are a few other food sources that can mess things up, too. Some people have very sensitive systems, and their hormones can easily be thrown off from these and other sources.

Stacey was one of those individuals with a sensitive system. We worked together for a few months, and in that time, she did notice some of her symptoms subsiding.

During a Skype session one day, Stacey told me, "My co-workers are so excited that I stopped turning the heat up in the office. I had no idea they were sweating all day since I was walking around with a sweater on. I did think it was a bit odd that my friend, Trina, was wearing sleeveless blouses in winter.

"I thought Trina was a little young to be having hot flashes," Stacey chuckled. "Little did I know it was me having chronic cold flashes. Anyway, I am so happy I'm not freezing to death anymore, but I still feel a little bloated and my weight loss has stalled."

I could sense Stacey was ready to take it to the next level. How about you? Are you ready to take it to the next level?

Another common cause of an underactive thyroid and/or the inability to shed those extra pounds, is from stress. When your body is at a high stress point all the time, it slows down your metabolism. As it sends in those little soldiers to fight, inflammation increases and weight loss is prevented. You will read more about stress reduction and why it is so important in the upcoming chapters.

If you are feeling symptoms like Stacey was, you will most likely benefit from a very gentle approach. By gentle, I mean removing certain foods from your daily intake that could be harming your system, and trying stress-relieving activities like yoga.

If your system is very sensitive, it might misinterpret certain foods as terrorists. The war I previously mentioned normally starts in your gut, and then spreads throughout the body.

The gut war can lead to inflammation, poor digestion, bloating, constipation, diarrhea, nausea, vomiting, GERD, diabetes, high blood pressure, and more.

When the body feels under attack, it will prevent weight loss, and might even trigger weight gain. The inflammation from the attack can even lead to rising blood sugar, blood pressure, and other diseases. If you have tried it all, but nothing is working, try this next step.

Since Stacey was still having some intestinal discomfort, I recommended cutting out some top allergen foods like dairy, eggs, and soy.

"Cut out dairy? You've got to be kidding me!" Stacey laughed. "I was tested for allergies a few years ago, and they didn't mention any food sensitivities. Come to think of it, I didn't test positive for gluten, but I do feel so much better now that I'm not eating it," she stated.

I shared with Stacey that it is common to have a food sensitivity without actually having a true allergy to it. In essence, the body still goes to war, but on a quieter, and less detectible level.

By the end of our session, Stacey decided she was ready to kick it up a notch. She was already avoiding gluten and drinking fluoride-free water. Over the next eight weeks, she avoided dairy, soy, and eggs. She replaced her morning protein shake with a non-dairy, vegan version (I recommend IsaLean non-dairy protein shakes and bars).

In the first few weeks, Stacey didn't feel much of a difference; but she continued the personalized plan I created for her. We discussed how it takes time for the body to heal before it can start letting go of the extra pounds.

At around week eight, Stacey started our session with an enormous smile. "I just can't believe it! I'm serious, I just can't believe it," Stacey beamed. "I don't understand how or why, but I'm finally not bloated anymore. My stomach is shrinking, my pants are loose, and my rings are even sliding around on my fingers. I think I must have been eating something before that was bugging my system. Ever since I cut that stuff out, I feel so much better. I have even started doing power yoga two days a week. My friends have noticed how much I have changed, and they want help, too. I told them to email you right away so they could get their own personalized plans."

I was so happy for Stacey. She was feeling better and headed toward her goal.

If you are like Stacey, and nothing you have tried is working, it may be an indication that a war is waging inside of you. It's time to stop that war and find a peaceful balance. When the body feels at peace, it can work like it was designed to.

As we have discussed, diet and lifestyle may have prompted nutrient deficiencies that are slowing everything down in your system. It is important to eliminate the source of the problems, but it is equally important to re-nourish the body to speed up the processes and get you feeling better.

The vitamins and supplements I recommend to rebalance the thyroid and rev up the metabolism are 4,000 iu of vitamin D; 200 mcg of selenium; 1 mg copper; and 20 mg of zinc per day. It's easy to get the recommended levels through a high quality multivitamin, and by enjoying lots of colorful vegetables.

In addition to your multivitamin, you can benefit from taking an adaptogen and probiotic supplement. Adaptogens are scientifically proven to lower stress levels, which will help you lose weight and feel great. I take mine every day, and it has been such a lifesaver. I refer to it as liquid gold, and always make sure to have it on hand.

Life is so much easier (and more fun) when you don't constantly feel stressed. Probiotics are another supplement that is vital in stopping and repairing the war in your gut. These little ambulances race around repairing the damage in our system.

Without these healers and peace keepers in our bodies, our hormones can be taken hostage by poor nutrition, lifestyle, and stress. Taking pure and clean probiotics, adaptogens, and multivitamins daily will catapult you toward feeling and looking amazing.

I take Isagenix Daily Essentials Multivitamins, Ionix Supreme adaptogens, and drink IsaLean protein shakes with probiotics every day.

To order your Isagenix supplements, contact us at www.thrivenutritionandfitness.com.

Chapter 16
Supplements: The Good, the Bad, and the Ugly

If we eat right, shouldn't we get all the nutrients we need from our food? I used to think so. So did my client, David.

"My parents never took vitamins, so why should I? If I'm eating healthier I should be fine," said David.

Supplements are not regulated by the Food and Drug Administration (FDA), and as such, I was hesitant to recommend any to my clients. Some of those vitamins we get from the grocery store could have anything in them – like dirt, bark, and other questionable things – even though they may be labeled "Vitamin C" or "Magnesium." Scary, right?

Over the years, our country has allowed the farming industry to overuse the soil and contaminate it with harmful pesticides and herbicides that kill all the nutrients. Surprisingly enough, healthy dirt actually has many vital nutrients that our bodies require to regulate our metabolisms. We should ingest these minerals by eating the plants that absorb the soil naturally during growth. However, in an effort to protect crops from pests, nutrient-killing chemicals have changed the healthy components of our topsoil, making those necessary minerals contaminated.

In efforts to grow plants faster to sell more crops, the growers also tend to use chemically-ridden fertilizers to speed up the process. The problem is that all this over-farming robs the soil of the necessary nutrients, and those nutrients are often replaced with unnatural chemicals. So if our food is lacking nutrients, then so are we.

A 2004 Landmark Study at the University of Texas established that six out of 13 general nutrients in fruits and vegetables had declined six to 38 percent over the past 50 years. Similar studies established that our plant-based foods contain about half the nutrient quantity they did 100 years ago.

The saddest part about the condition of our soils, is the end product. Although these fruits and vegetables are void of quality nutrients, they may look the same (if not better) than produce grown without pesticides and other chemicals. As consumers, we often choose the "pretty" produce, unaware that it is deficient in vitamins and minerals, and coated in disease-causing chemicals.

When David asked me about the necessity of supplements in a healthy diet, I asked him about the quality of the produce he was eating. I went on to explain to him the differences between non-organic (conventional) and organic fruits and vegetables. It is rather shocking what pesticides are doing to our bodies.

Do you know where pesticides originated from? They did not even come into existence until after World War II. Scientists made an accidental discovery that the neurological gases they were using during warfare, were killing bugs. So, they decided to knock the potency down a few notches and spray it on farm crops to keep the bugs from eating them. That's right! I said they are spraying neurologically poisonous gases on our fruits and vegetables to keep the bugs at bay. That is why I recommend eating organic produce. Leave the conventional produce behind!

My family has a garden year-round to help keep the grocery bill down. In the winter, we grow broccoli, cauliflower, romaine and other lettuces. Most of these grow well into the spring. In the summer, we grow tomatoes, zucchini, squash, beans, peppers, and eggplant. The fall brings the planting of carrots, squash, and more tomatoes. Whether you have a big garden or just a few pots on the patio, growing your own food cuts grocery bills down. When we grow more than we can eat, we freeze it for later.

Eating organically is helpful, but it is still difficult to consume every little vitamin and mineral our bodies need on a daily basis. In that regard, I do recommend taking a few supplements; and those recommendations are pretty individualized. Scheduling a session with a Board Certified Registered Dietitian is best.

As a general rule, I recommend starting off with a high quality daily multivitamin. Also, it is often helpful to add an Omega 3 supplement. If you are not a fan of vegetables or are not getting enough, I also recommend pure and natural powdered greens.

For more information on supplements, contact us at www.ThriveNutritionandFitness.com.

By the end of my session with David, he had already placed his order for a Men's daily vitamin, Omega 3s, powdered greens, and a supplement for energy and stress reduction. Five days later I got an email from him.

"I can't believe how much better I feel. I have the energy to lift weights after work, and I feel like I can handle life a little better. The small stuff that use to get me all fired up isn't bothering me as much. My wife and coworkers are even noticing the difference. I had no idea how bad I was feeling since that was how I always felt. Thank you for telling me about these products. Between these and eating better, I feel like I can take on the world," said David.

Everyone's results may vary, but David's reaction is commonly the feedback I receive. Even with a healthy diet, there can still be vitamin and mineral gaps, which is why supplements are so helpful.

Whatever supplement you decide to try, be extremely careful. If it isn't third party tested or contains fillers and oxidized oils – like most sold over the counter – do not take them. They can cause more problems than benefits, including the increase of systemic inflammation, and prevention of weight loss.

Chapter 17
Last Call For Happy Hour

Do you tend to wind down each day with a glass or two of your favorite alcoholic beverage? In today's world, it is common to feel so stressed out that we turn to food or alcohol to decompress from the day. Many of my clients work full time, have long commutes, and have extensive family responsibilities. All these demands can be physically, mentally, and emotionally draining. That is why your body is waiving a white flag each evening saying, "Help! The stress is too much. I need comfort."

Often times when we feel like this, it's easy to grab that bottle of booze and drink our worries away. Although it might help you relax at that moment in time, it is wreaking havoc on your body and your metabolism. It is important to comfort our bodies and intentionally take part in destressing activities daily. We will cover this more in PART III, NOURISH YOUR SOUL.

Alcohol is actually a toxin that clogs up the liver. When the liver is busy processing alcohol, it cannot regulate the blood sugar as well as it usually does. This causes the body to leave the fat-burning mode and go into the fat-storing mode. This, in turn, slows down the metabolism by up to 30 percent! It's like driving along at 60 mph, and quickly braking down to 40 mph. If you are trying to reach your weight loss goals, this is not helpful.

Fancy cocktails also contain a lot of empty calories in the alcohol and mixers. Hard liquor is about 100 calories per ounce, and it turns straight into body fat. Say you combine that with a common margarita mix, and your sugar consumption shoots up to about 14 teaspoons per drink. Yikes!

Most mixed drinks are loaded in sugar. The average person would have to walk about six miles to burn off one mixed drink. Maybe sugary drinks are not your thing, but you enjoy beer or wine. Yes, they are lower in sugar, but they still contain harmful ingredients. Beer is made from grain, so it has inflammatory-causing gluten as an ingredient – and it's also high in carbohydrates. Wine isn't that much better. Made from grapes, it is high in sugar and carbs.

You would have to walk a mile for each 12-ounce beer, or six-ounce glass of wine, just to burn off the sugar from them. I'm not saying to you can never indulge again, but if you are serious about losing weight, it will be incredibly helpful to cut out the alcohol. How can we expect to look and feel better if we put toxins and poisons in our bodies?

If you still feel the need to have an occasional drink, I recommend sticking with a clear spirit like vodka, and limiting your portions to one or two ounces. If spirits aren't your thing, you may enjoy a hard cider. Since they are made from fruit, they don't contain gluten, and they even have a low-sugar "light" option available.

Whatever you decide, remember to limit your portions. From years of experience in helping others, I have seen alcohol being the one thing that has held people back.

Chapter 18
Needs Beyond Food

News Flash: Your Body Is Talking. Are You Listening? Just like all other animals, we have needs. There are the physical necessities, like breathing, eating, sleeping, and the need for intimacy and safety. We also have the emotional needs of being loved, feeling a sense of belonging, and friendship. These physical and emotional essentials help us develop our interpretation of loving and respecting ourselves and others.

When all of these needs are met, we become free to be more spontaneous and courageous, and we are the most effective at being ourselves. You may know this theory as Maslow's Hierarchy of Human Needs. Research has proven that we require these needs to be tended to, or our systems do not work at the optimal level we expect them to each day.

The first step in creating a healthy lifestyle, is to start listening to your body. This can be very difficult at first. Over the years, I have met so many clients that look at me totally lost and bewildered when I first ask them, "What is your body telling you? How do you feel physically? What does your body need?"

These questions may sound strange to us as adults. We are often so busy caring for others, that we ignore our own physical needs. Who has time for that? If you feel like this, you are not alone. Our society has taught us to be too busy. Even I have found myself filling up all the available time in my calendar in an effort to be productive. We have been trained to stay busy, lest we be called "lazy."

Have you ever found yourself skipping meals because, "you are just too busy?" Unfortunately, this is very common these days. But if you stop and think about it, would you skip breathing because you are just too busy? Of course not. So why do we force our bodies to continue activities without feeding them? It's like expecting your car to take you to work with no gas in the tank. We tend to use and abuse our bodies, and then become surprised and upset when they give out on us.

Maybe you have been wanting to lose weight for years, or get your blood pressure and blood sugar under control, but there never seems to be enough time. Well, you may be right. If we allow other activities, like work, families, or even church, to become a priority over caring for ourselves, they will. Life will get in the way of survival, if you let it.

We all have a mountain of responsibilities looking down on us each day, but how can we take care of business if we don't take the time to take care of ourselves? If we want our bodies to improve, setting aside the time to care for them must be a priority.

Prepare for Success, and You Are Likely to Succeed

It is inevitable. We are going to get hungry multiple times each day. If we are not ready, the hunger monster will strike. As our blood sugars start to dip, our bodies send out a hunger hormone called ghrelin, to signal us to eat. So what happens when we are too busy to eat? Our ghrelin levels increase until our bodies are screaming at us. At this point, survival instincts kick in, and we grab the first thing in sight. Maybe it's fast food, or chips from the vending machine. Whatever the choice is, it usually doesn't leave us feeling very well. The trick is to be prepared, and stay ahead of the game.

Before we can prepare food, we must first make sure we have food to prepare. I often start by pulling out a few recipes my family likes. It's fun to try at least one new recipe each week. This helps keep eating fun and interesting. Maybe one week you feel like Thai food, and try a new Pad Thai chicken over spaghetti squash (instead of noodles). The next week, maybe you feel like trying a new Italian or Mexican recipe. It is important to mix it up.

Try recipes with bold or interesting flavors. Utilizing herbs, spices, garlic, onions, and peppers is a great way to add a ton of flavor and nutrients. Strong flavors such as garlic or spices, send signals to the brain that we are being nourished. The brain then starts sending out a hormone called leptin, which tells us we are not hungry anymore, so we can stop eating.

Once I have four to five recipes picked out, I make a list. I check the fridge and pantry to see what items I need for dinner recipes, as well as other staples we need to get us through the week. I usually add one to two servings of fruit per person, Greek yogurt, string cheese, organic milk, a variety of vegetables, and so forth. I've also learned to make that list while I'm at home, otherwise it's inevitable that I'll forget a vital ingredient.

Making a list not only keeps me on track, but it also helps to keep grocery bills down. And just before I go to the store, I grab a snack. Ever shop on an empty stomach? It's not pretty. And it's a sure-fire way to end up with way more than I need.

I do normally double-up on the meat for one or two of the recipes. We find it can be incredibly efficient to always have a few leftovers on hand. If time is running short, warming up those leftovers and adding in a few vegetables can have dinner ready in a few minutes time.

What about lunches? You know you are probably going to be busy at work, or find yourself running late in the morning. The best way to be prepared each day, is to pack a lunch and snacks the night before. I cannot stress this enough. Even if I am working from home, I make a mental note after dinner of what I am going to enjoy the next day. Often I make extra at dinner, and pack the leftovers in separate containers to be enjoyed as lunch in the days to follow.

Don't let the hunger monster sneak up on you. Take a few minutes to enjoy your mid-morning snack. Maybe fruit and nuts, or Greek yogurt. Make the time to leave your desk for snacks and lunches. Mentally, it can be so refreshing to step away from work for a few minutes. I often find myself taking a short five to ten-minute walk outside during snack time.

It is also very important to focus on actually enjoying your meal. Leave the computer, iPad, and phone alone during this time. Eating while distracted can leave you feeling like you didn't eat at all. Your brain works best focusing on one task at a time. So when eating, try to focus on the way the food looks, smells, tastes, and feels in your mouth. Slow down during meal time. It takes our bodies about fifteen minutes to stop producing our hunger hormone, ghrelin, and start producing our fullness hormone, leptin.

Eating should be enjoyable, so please slow down and take the time to enjoy it. You may notice that you actually feel full much sooner than you have in the past. Once you start feeling satisfied, your body signals that it has sufficient energy (so there is no need to keep eating).

Some people like to rate their hunger on a scale of 1 to 10, with one being starving, and ten being stuffed. Remember, we should start eating when we are just starting to get hungry, around a hunger scale of three or four, and stop eating when we are just starting to get full, around a hunger scale of six.

Sleep

Some people need more sleep than others, but there is no questions that we all need it. The American Sleep Association recommends getting seven to nine hours of quality sleep every night. During sleep, our bodies can focus on repairing cells and growing new cells. Since our bodies are constantly being exposed to stress and pollutants, we are in constant need of repair.

Many people try to function on four or five hours of sleep, but they often notice new problems arising. This was the case for Robert, a retired firefighter with a bad back. His main concern was to lose weight, because he knew the excess was causing his back pain to get worse. Over the months, Robert learned how the wrong carbohydrates were increasing inflammation in his body and making his pain worse, so he cut back. He also was open to changing from non-fat foods, to whole foods with heart-healthy fats. We adjusted his nutrition significantly over time, but Robert continued to have difficulty losing weight and controlling his hunger.

During one session, Robert mentioned not sleeping well. He often watched TV and surfed the Internet until about 2 a.m., since he didn't feel sleepy. We went on to discuss the effects of the blue light emitted from electronic devices, and how this light stimulates our brains. It also decreases our body's natural ability to produce our sleep hormone, melatonin.

Robert also mentioned that the shows he watched were action-packed, which reminded him of his days as a fire captain. Although he enjoyed the shows, he determined that they may be part of what was keeping him awake and leaving him feeling so tired and hungry the next day.

We went on to chat about how being tired can decrease our desire to make healthy choices, and can cause us to eat more. On a subconscious level, we may feel like the food will give us more energy. But instead, we often choose high carbohydrate options which just cause us to feel more tired.

By the end of the session, Robert had decided to turn electronics off by 10 p.m., and then read or draw until he felt sleepy. After a few weeks, his body was able to produce melatonin earlier, allowing him to fall asleep faster.

Later, Robert shared with me that he noticed it was easier to make healthier food choices and eat for true hunger, since he wasn't so tired anymore. Getting more sleep allowed Robert's back to heal faster, and he was able to shed those extra pounds he had been trying to get rid of for years.

If you are having problems falling or staying asleep, be sure to limit or avoid naps after 2 p.m. If you do nap, limit it to an hour or less. Often, a 30-minute power nap can be most effective for getting you through the remainder of your day, but not invade your sleep at night. Another helpful tip is to make sure you are getting in enough physical movement during the day. Our bodies are meant to move, so don't spend all day sitting, or your body may have difficulty falling asleep at night.

It can be helpful to get a pedometer, and aim for seven to ten thousand steps each day. This sounds like a lot, but it can easily be accomplished by getting in an extra hour of walking daily. Maybe you walk a quick mile on your lunch break, and take a stroll after dinner. My kids love putting on fun music and dancing around after dinner, or going on a "nature walk." Do whatever you need to do to get moving. Find something you enjoy, and do it daily.

If you are not having restful sleep, make sure to remember your evening snack. A common myth is to stop eating after 6:00 p.m., but that can actually slow down your metabolism and cause blood sugar crashes during the night. Instead, controlling carbohydrate portions at dinner and snacking before bed will keep blood sugar stable and promote restful sleep.

We normally eat dinner between 5 and 6 p.m., and have a snack at around 9 p.m. It's important to avoid sugary snacks before bed, since they will cause blood sugar to skyrocket, and then crash. Instead, aim to have a half cup of fruit with a healthy fat. I love apple slices and nut butter, or baby carrots and avocado dip. The small amount of sugar in the fruit and vegetables prevents bottoming out blood sugars, and the healthy fat slows digestion to promote stable blood sugars. This all supports restful sleep, so you can wake feeling refreshed and ready to tackle the day. Don't underestimate the importance of sleep. Cherish it and protect it.

Hydrate

It's no secret that one of the best things we can do for our body is drink lots of good, clean water. In fact, fluid needs are higher than previously thought. We need 90 to 120 ounces per day to maintain adequate hydration.

The body is made up of about 66% water, but fluid losses occur continuously through urination, evaporation through the skin, and even breathing. Additional losses occur when the climate is warmer, and during exercise.

Drinking water helps to protect our organs, and helps flush out toxins in the body. Since our skin is the largest organ we have, it requires lots of water. Adequate hydration will support healthy, nourished skin. Inadequate hydration can lead to dry, cracked skin, leaving us open to an increased risk of infection.

As a bonus, proper hydration decreases food cravings, and helps us to feel full, longer. In order to maintain good health, fluid levels must be replaced to avoid dehydration.

At times we feel signals from our bodies that we need something, but we don't know what it is. Often times, we eat in an effort to restore internal order and quench that feeling. The problem is, that we may just be thirsty, so eating doesn't resolve the issue. This can lead to more eating, because we can't shake the feeling. The next time you feel like this, ask yourself when you last ate, and how much water you drank. If you have eaten recently – and you are not feeling hunger signals (discussed in previous chapters) – then odds are your body is requesting fluids.

It is said that if you become thirsty, you are actually dehydrated. Drinking water throughout the day before you start to thirst can help your body function smoothly. Dehydration can actually become a dangerous situation, and at the very least, make you feel tired, weak and irritable. It can also cause you to feel hungry and trigger over-eating, diminishing your ability to burn calories effectively, and lower your metabolism. So, drink up!

If plain, old-fashioned water doesn't wet your whistle, try adding a few slices of lemon, lime, apple, or peach; or how about some muddled berries and fresh mint? It's not only delicious, but you'll gain a few extra nutrients without a lot of calories or additives.

Tea is a great option, too. Green tea is loaded with catechins - potent antioxidants - and a small amount of natural caffeine. The combination of catechins and caffeine can increase metabolic rate, helping you burn more calories. Green tea can also help decrease systemic inflammation and detoxify the body. Studies show that the effects are increased by the potency of the tea, so use two tea bags (or twice as much loose tea) per cup, and aim for two cups per day. Green tea is also best when brewed at 180 degrees Fahrenheit, for three to five minutes (any longer will make the tea more bitter).

Sweeten your tea with a squeeze of orange, a few mashed berries, or a sprinkle of stevia. And be sure to enjoy your caffeinated teas before 2 p.m. for optimum sleep at night. After that, switch to water, fruit-flavored water, or decaffeinated herbal teas.

Slow Down and Breathe

Do you find yourself hurrying from task to task throughout the day? Most of us do. Maybe your mornings involve racing around the house trying to get ready for work, thinking about the busy day you have, and everything you need to get done. As soon as you get yourself dressed, it's a sprint out the door in an effort to beat the morning traffic. Just when you think you made it on the road in time, you get caught behind the slowest truck ever. Your thoughts then speed up as the traffic slows down, and now you're worried about walking in to work late.

Does this sound familiar? Your mind is spinning and you haven't even made it to the office yet! Day to day stress can be overwhelming. This high-anxiety environment can cause us to take quick, shallow breaths, which increases the stress in our bodies. Our brains start releasing cortisol - that dreaded stress hormone - because our thoughts and breaths are sending signals to our bodies that we need to go into survival mode.

Think back to a time when our ancestors were hunters and gatherers. It was an era of hunting and being hunted. When being chased by a wild animal, they either faced them and fought, or ran away as fast as they could — Fight or Flight. In order to stay alive, the body needed those stress signals to go into survival mode. Fear and stress coupled with fast, shallow breathing usually signaled a life and death situation.

Today, our bodies still have those instincts ingrained in us. So when we are in a high-stress situation (subconsciously taking quick, shallow breaths), our bodies go into that survival mode. The brain releases cortisol, and we start storing energy instead of using it. Feeling overwhelmed and stressed out can cause us to gain weight and feel totally wiped out.

Since we can't change our genetic makeup, it is important to manage our stress levels. One of the best ways is to slow down and take a few deep breaths. Deep breathing releases tension from the body and clears the mind, improving both physical and mental wellness. Taking a few deep breaths also causes the body to feel more relaxed. The body senses an improved situation and stops releasing cortisol. In a more relaxed state, the body resumes burning calories instead of storing them.

Nancy is a perfect example of Fight or Flight. I had been seeing her for a little while, and she was making progress. And then that progress slowed way down.

Nancy was a single mother (and grandmother), working full-time. She was constantly in a state of trying to juggle all her responsibilities. During a telephone session one day, she shared with me how her stress level was stuck at full throttle; she was feeling like she couldn't get enough oxygen.

After listening to her situation, I started asking Nancy a series of questions. She was sticking pretty closely to her personalized nutrition plan; she was also sleeping fairly well at night. She just couldn't seem to take a deep breath. That was my clue.

For the rest of the session, I shared with Nancy the research behind breathing, and how it can change the chemistry of the body. Since she was craving oxygen, she was open to the idea of intentional deep breathing. After all, it was something she could do anywhere.

Nancy started using some time on her commute to work to turn off the radio and focus on slowing down her breathing. After taking a few deep breaths, she noticed she could think more clearly. Using this technique when she was feeling stressed, helped her days go a bit more smoothly. Soon, Nancy was making a mindful effort to schedule ten to 15 minutes, a few times a day, to focus on deep breathing. She did it on her commute to and from work, and before bed. To her amazement, her pants started getting loser and her energy level was rising.

Over the next few months, Nancy met her goal weight. She continues to make time in her day for daily breathing exercises; she has even taught the techniques to her children and grandchildren. It's a great way to naturally decrease stress and tension, and it doesn't cost you anything.

When breathing, the importance of good posture cannot be overstated. While sitting, we tend to slouch. This compresses the diaphragm and other organs, resulting in shallow breathing. Slouching also strains muscles in the neck and back. It is helpful to sit in a chair with good back support to avoid the fatigue that leads to slouching.

How To Do Deep Breathing:

1. Sit up straight (do not arch your back).
2. Exhale completely through your mouth.
3. Place your hands on your stomach, just above your waist.
4. Breathe in slowly through your nose, extending your hands out with your stomach - this ensures that you are breathing deeply (imagine you are filling your body with air from the bottom up).
5. Breathe in for a slow count of four. Hold for one second. Exhale for a count of four.
6. Repeat for several minutes.

After you get some experience, you don't need to use your hands to check your breathing.

You can also practice deep breathing exercises lying on your back, standing up, sitting in traffic, in line at the store, etc. Deep breathing exercises can help you to relax before you go to sleep for the night, fall back asleep if you awaken in the middle of the night, or anytime you are feeling really tense or short of breath. Simply concentrate on slowly breathing in and out.

Remember...slow down and BREATHE!

Exercise

"I just don't get it. I have been working out at the gym for an hour, five days a week. I wake up at 4:30 each morning to get my workout in, and spend the weekends chasing my grandkids. I am burning more calories, but not losing weight. I thought maybe I wasn't trying hard enough, so I added in an evening spin class three days a week, and a kickboxing class on two other days. What the heck? Why can't I lose a single pound?" said Bonnie.

Why Can't I Lose Weight?

Although I had just met Bonnie, I have heard her story all too frequently. Actually, as a lover of cardio, I could relate. Cardio exercises like running, spin classes, and kickboxing are fun at the time. All that cardio releases endorphins in the brain to make us feel better. And those endorphins can become addicting.

The problem with all this cardio, is it causes us to take fast, shallow breaths, and triggers the brain to think we are being chased by that wild animal again. The cardio can cause a downpour of cortisol from our brain, increasing stress hormones. The body feels the need to go into survival mode, and starts storing energy instead of burning it. Even though the treadmill or heart rate monitor may say you have burned a ton of calories, if you are forcing your body into fat-storing mode, then the calories burned are not helping. The next time you eat, the body is going to store those calories in preparation for a shortage.

I am a fan of cardio, too, but if your goal is to lose weight and decrease your stress levels, you will need to limit it. As a former half-marathoner, this was not easy for me. But the more I transitioned into weightlifting, the stronger I felt. As with anything, a great rule is balance.

I recommend limiting cardio to about 30 minutes per session, and including interval training in those workouts. Studies show that varying intensities during a workout helps you burn more calories – and you continue burning more calories after the workout is over. So hit that interval button on the treadmill; or try moving at a slow pace for two minutes, increase your speed for two minutes, go all out for 30 to 60 seconds, and then go back down to your initial pace. By varying your pace, you are varying your heart rate. This allows time for you to take a few deep breaths - and prevent that cortisol from being released.

Resistance training - or weightlifting - is another very important component of your workout. Whether you use your own body weight, free weights, resistance bands, or machines, it is important to get in a few days of resistance exercise each week.

Resistance exercise builds muscle and protects bone health. Without resistance exercise, our muscles become unable to protect our bones and we increase the risk of breaks and fractures. I recommend starting with body weight resistance exercises, like squats, lunges, sit-ups and push-ups. These are great because they can be done anywhere (at home in your pajamas, or on your lunch break at the office). Once you feel comfortable, you may like to challenge yourself more by adding in some free weights. I love using a kettle ball, because it's one piece of equipment I can use for all kinds of great exercises.

Bonnie was blown away by the information we discussed. She couldn't believe that all this cardio could actually be stalling her weight loss. She was so happy to hear that sleep was more important than killing herself at the gym, and decided to switch up her workouts.

I recommended varying between a HIIT (High Intensity Interval Training) workout and yoga, a few days a week. A HIIT workout can be done anywhere - like at home or at a gym – and you can find all kinds of interesting options on YouTube and Pinterest. HIIT workouts range from beginners (using only your body weight) to advanced (using free weights); and they are perfect for almost everyone. It's a great way to get the right combination of cardio and resistance efficiently, and keep you in the calorie burning mode.

Yoga is another great way to move our bodies. The stretching, deep breathing, and calm environment is a great way to release the day's tension, while getting in a great workout. So many of us sit during the day, and our bodies can start to contract and ache. Yoga is a great remedy for this.

During one of our sessions, I asked Bonnie how her average workday went. As she guided me through her day, I noticed that she was sitting for an hour on her commute to and from work; sitting at her desk for eight or nine hours; sitting for 30 minutes at lunch (and again at dinner each night); and finally, she was sitting from 8 to 10 p.m. while she watched her favorite television shows. Bonnie was sitting for 13 to 14 hours a day! And all that sitting was causing her hips and back to ache.

I asked Bonnie how she felt about yoga, and she said that she was "probably too old to be bending like that." You may have similar thoughts if it is something you haven't tried before. But Bonnie was in enough pain to give it a try. I recommended that she start with a beginner's class, or even a DVD.

After a few sessions, Bonnie shared with me that she had found a "hot" yoga class that helped her hips and back tremendously. The heat helped her relax and stretch her muscles. But more than the stretching, she loved making time for herself to do something that she enjoyed. The peaceful environment helped calm her mind. The stretching helped extend her body so that it didn't ache anymore.

After six months of working together with Bonnie, she was well on her way toward her goal weight and feeling better than ever. Changing up her workout routine helped her lose weight and tone up. Now, she does a HIIT workout for 30 minutes, three days a week, and yoga a few days a week. Bonnie reports feeling more strength, energy, and balance than ever before.

PART III
NOURISH YOUR SOUL

Chapter 19
Thank Your Lucky Stars

Even though life is not perfect, we are so blessed with the things that we have. It can be easy to look around, and think that we need more. Maybe our cars or clothes are not as nice as the Jones'; or perhaps we don't have the means to take fancy vacations like some. But we have been gifted with blessings that are much more valuable than material things.

Let me start off by sharing my gratitude to live in America, where we are free to choose our religion, profession, beliefs, and much more. We all too often forget about these blessings, because they are just part of our normal life - but they are so vital to us! In other countries, it is against the law for women to go to school (let alone get a degree), or practice nutritional counseling, or even write a book. It is easy to take everyday life for granted.

I am reminded of our blessings every time I turn on the news. It seems like there is always someone dying of an incurable disease, being shot at, or just going without. If you wake up with air in your lungs, food to eat, a bed to sleep on, and a roof over your head, be thankful.

"Every day I wake up above ground, I am thankful," said George, who was referred to me by his doctor. George has a chronic disease that could take his life. Despite the fact that he had lost his left leg, as well as the sight from his right eye because of this illness, he was determined to improve the health in the rest of his body.

George always showed up to each virtual session early, along with his caregiver to take notes for him.

"It would be easy for me to give up. It would be easy to just sit in that wheelchair all day and let my life pass me by. But for some reason, I feel like I still have something to offer this world. For some reason, God has spared my life and I feel the need to give back for as long as can. I just figure every day is a blessing and I am going to give it all I have for as long as I have," George told me during our first session together. I could tell he was a fighter, with the gift of looking at his life as a "glass half full."

Every session, George and I would review his nutrition and fitness routine. He shared how he would bike a few miles on his stationary bike, and then move on to weightlifting each day. Each session would end with stretching and prayer, thanking God for the gift of the day.

Even though George only had one good leg and one good eye, he still went to the local food bank to volunteer a few days each week. To this day, George makes me so aware of all the blessings bestowed on me.

It is helpful to start each day with the intentional habit of being thankful for all the blessings in your life. Your body may not be perfect, but it has blessed you in so many ways. It enables you to live, eat, work, and love those you care for most. Your legs may not be as long or lean as your friend's, but they still carry you around this beautiful earth. Don't have a six pack? Those abs you have still protect the organs that keep you alive. Even if your arms are not as toned as you would like them to be, they can still give someone a hug that can change their day for the better. Love what you have.

Chapter 20
Pencil In Some "ME TIME"

If you feel like your days are a constant race to the finish line, you are not alone. That is how most of my clients feel - like the years are passing them by. If you can't remember what you did yesterday, then you may be suffering from a "QVQ Life" (quantity vs. quality). I have this habit, too. I just naturally try to pack in way too much, in too little time. It drives my husband nuts. Actually, it drives me nuts as well.

If you can relate, and find yourself always at a hectic pace, then stop. Even though it seems crazy, we actually have control over our own schedules. If you feel stressed and burnt out, it may be related to constantly overbooking yourself. Everything in life is a choice. We don't have to get out of bed and go to work each morning. Nobody is making us. We choose to do it, because there are consequences (like paying the bills and other responsibilities). I keep looking for that money tree, but haven't found it yet. So, how do we manage the chaos?

It can be helpful to use a Day Planner, and write out your exact routine in pencil for the week. Next, highlight all the activities needed to sustain life, like eating, sleeping, and working (so you have a place to eat and sleep). Then review all the activities you do, such as a morning devotional, watching television, social media, shopping, etc. Do all of these activities improve your life? Are they helping you obtain your health and weight loss goals? If the answer is NO, erase them. For the purpose of this exercise, don't think about it, just do it.

Now, how much time do you have left in your week? If you are like most of us, you may realize how much time is spent on negative activities that are holding you back from your goals. The average American spends three hours each day watching television. Maybe you didn't realize that you were spending 21 hours each week watching the Food Network or HGTV. No wonder there was no time to work out or prep meals.

Perhaps you found you were spending 30 minutes a day driving through fast food places because you were rushed. If you added that time up, could it have been spent at that HIIT or yoga class you've been wanting to try but never found the time? After erasing unnecessary activities, you may be blown away by the time available in your schedule. Making time to care for yourself is vital to survival. If you don't do it, no one else is going to.

Next, write in an activity that makes you feel relaxed, for 20 minutes each day. It is a great idea to do this around the time of day that you are feeling the most stress. Are your mornings crazy? Then take 20 minutes to calm and center yourself. You are worth the time. Similarly, if you find that your stress level is highest in the evenings, and you feel burnt out, schedule your "Me Time" for the end of the day.

"Me Time" activities are things you can do easily, that make you feel empowered, strengthened, or relaxed. Examples are prayer, meditation, yoga, taking a walk, weightlifting, talking to a good friend, crafting, or reading an inspirational book. This time is devoted to rebuilding and refreshing you. It's only 20 minutes out of a 24-hour day, so no excuses. You are worth it.

After you have scheduled in your daily self-care activities, then write in things that you choose to do to help others. It may be taking the kids to sports, caring for a family member, or volunteering at church. Caring for others is important to nourish the soul, but should not come before caring for yourself. After all, how can you care for others, if you neglect yourself or run yourself into the ground?

Last, but not least, let's talk about the word, "NO." Everything is a choice, and that means we have the choice - and the responsibility - to sometimes say no.

I asked my client, Shannon, what was preventing her from getting in her "Me Time." She had the classic answer that her life was so busy between work and family, that there was not any time left in the day for her. It is all too easy to feel like that, especially when caring for others is your responsibility.

I asked Shannon if she felt like she was providing the best care possible to her family. That's when the tears started to flow. I could hear her getting choked up. After a long pause, she firmly said, "No. I have been short with my kids and husband. I plan outings with my friends, but I can't even enjoy them because I am so worried I will be late to the next appointment I planned that day."

When I asked Shannon if she felt balanced, she said, "Not at all! I feel like I am juggling ten balls in the air and any one of them could fall at any time. I hate it."

For homework, I asked Shannon to complete the weekly schedule activity. She reluctantly agreed, but said, "You don't understand. If I don't do all these things, no one else will."

I told Shannon that I did understand, and had felt like that too. I also noticed that the more responsibilities I took on, the more I was given (and the more miserable I became). Feeling relieved that she was not alone, Shannon agreed to complete the weekly scheduling exercise.

At our next session, Shannon was excited to share that she had scheduled in Me Time for eight o'clock each night, after she put the kids to bed. We chatted about how that was working.

"Some days it works, and some days it doesn't, because I get busy working on the books I have to do for my husband's company," said Shannon. I asked her how she felt on days she was successful, and what she was doing for her self-care activity. Shannon shared that she felt better, slept better, and was nicer to her family when she got her yoga in. When she didn't, she noticed she was snippier.

I asked Shannon which way she wanted to feel. "Of course I want to feel better, and be nicer to my family. I hate it when I snap at them. I guess this means that if I want to feel better and act nicer, then I need to get in my Me Time every day. It's best for everyone. I can't believe I just said that! It's best for me and my family when I make time for myself; I'm a better mom, wife, and person."

I could hear Shannon crying again, and I knew this was really sinking in. I asked her why she thought she felt better after taking some time for herself.

"I think it's because it's like drawing a line in the sand. It's me taking a stand for myself. It tells me that I am important. That I am worth the time. Walking or yoga makes me feel strong and empowered. I stand taller, and am proud to know that I am worth it," said Shannon.

Weeks later, Shannon had scheduled in her Me Time each day. She shifted other responsibilities around her self-care. When her friends asked her to volunteer for the school bake off, she checked her schedule first instead of just always saying yes. If she knew that it was going to be a crazy week with work and kids sports, she politely declined. To her surprise, the other moms stepped up and made more than enough.

Shannon noticed, "For the first time, I realized I don't have to do it all. Maybe I was holding someone else back before because I was doing everything. I'm going to say no a little more often now. It's not going to be the end of the world if I can't juggle everything. Someone else will help, they have so far."

By cutting down on surfing social media and asking her family to help get the kids to sports, Shannon was able to get in time to grocery shop, prep meals and snacks, workout three times a week, and get in her 20 minutes of Me Time each day. After six months, she had lost over 30 pounds and was happier than ever before.

Sometimes we feel that life is so busy, it's just passing us by. When that happens, get out your planner and start erasing those time-stealing, negative activities, and make more time for self-care. Use that Me Time to relax, and strengthen your heart, mind and soul. Give yourself permission to care for yourself.

Making this happen can change your life and will nourish your soul. After all, why put so much effort into not being able to enjoy your life. Slow down. Spend more quality time with yourself, and others that you love.

Don't let life pass you by.

Chapter 21
Quiet Your Mind, Feed Your Soul
Prayer and Meditation

"It all seems so overwhelming at times," shared Tom. "I am trying so hard to do all the right things, but my health is still not as good as I want it to be. To top it off, now my work is moving me to a new department. I just don't think I can keep this up."

Do you relate to Tom? I know I do. Sometimes life can feel so out of control that it is mentally and emotionally exhausting. Tom shared with me that he had been feeling so tired that he stopped going for daily walks, and was picking up fast food more often. He was feeling emotionally exhausted from thinking about all the change that was occurring in his life.

Some of the change was in his control: He wanted to change his nutrition and fitness habits. But some of it was out of his control, like his department change at work. Feeling a loss of control can be overwhelming and exhausting, but it is helpful to take a step back and remember that we are not in control as much as we think. We can get stuck in traffic on the way to work, forget to take our lunch, or (heaven forbid) get in an accident.

If we take a step back, it can actually be a relief to consider the fact that while we may have plans, they don't necessarily determine our destiny. Life went on before us, and will go on after us. It's our responsibility to do the best we can in the moment at hand.

Studies show that taking a mental health break using prayer or meditation actually lowers our stress levels. By now, we know that lower stress levels equal lower blood sugar, blood pressure, and body weight. Not to mention, we feel a whole lot better when we aren't totally stressed out.

Some people dedicate a room in their house to nothing but prayer or meditation, but you don't have to. I have a place in my family room that I feel at peace. So when the house is quiet in the morning, I sit on the couch with my daily devotional and read. Sometimes I don't feel like reading, so I stretch and focus on handing over my problems to God. After all, it's all His plan. You can do this verbally, or speak with the voice of your mind – whatever is most comfortable. Just find a few minutes each day to let go of the troubles. Taking a mental and emotional health break can renew and refresh your mind, body and soul. For me, it's incredibly calming to know that this is all part of God's plan.

If you are not religious, you can find similar relief through meditation. Meditation, or focusing on one thought or object, is like taking a mental health break from life. In the yoga world, some people chant, "ohm," while they meditate and stretch. Verbally saying the word focuses your mind away from chaos. The actual meaning behind ohm, is that some believe the universe creates a constant humming sound, and chanting this word unifies one with the energy of the universe. Any way you look at it, saying a word over and over is distracting you from other thoughts.

There are lots of ways to meditate. You can use visual meditation by lighting a candle, or looking at a picture of a scenic view. Focusing your thoughts on that object for a set amount of time can be just as effective.

Meditation is great because it is something you can do in an office. Try framing a picture of a scenic view from a vacation you went on, or would like to go on. During your break each day, focus on the picture. What would it feel like to be there? Would the weather be warm? How would the sun feel on your skin? What would you be thinking if you were there? How would you feel if you were there? If your mind starts to wonder, just let the thought go like a wave in the ocean, and return your focus to the picture.

Scientific studies show that prayer or meditation for 15 minutes each day drastically lowers stress and anxiety levels. It can boost your mood, and leave you feeling more in control of the tasks at hand. Feeling refreshed and in control can boost productivity toward your goals.

I shared this information with Tom, and asked him to try it. He responded by saying that he use to do this each morning and it did help him feel better. He couldn't even remember why he stopped, but he was willing to start again.

"I'll start tomorrow morning. I'll set my alarm 20 minutes early, and do it as soon as I get out of bed. I like to sit at the kitchen table, since that is where I can watch the sun come up," said Tom.

By our next session, Tom noticed he was feeling more comfortable with the changes occurring in his life. He said that the changes did not determine who he was as a person, they were merely variations in his environment. This sense of comfort with himself increased his mental and emotional strength.

"It feels like putting on a suit of armor each morning. As long as I have on my mental armor, no one can hurt my soul if I don't let them. It makes me feel so much stronger as a person. People at work are telling me I look happier, and my weightlifting partner has even been surprised. It's amazing how much more I can do at the gym when I feel stronger on the inside," Tom said in our session.

Tom is a perfect example of how important it is to nourish your mind, body, and especially your soul. When we strengthen our souls and grow belief in ourselves, our minds and bodies gain strength.

I invite you to schedule in 20 minutes each day to strengthen your soul.

Chapter 22
Laughter Is the Best Medicine

Laughter is a fundamental part of everyday life. Whether you are laughing at your child making silly faces, at a coworker telling a joke, or at a funny television show, laughter really is the best medicine. It's a universal language we subconsciously learn and share with every culture.

Laughter has emotional as well as physical benefits. It lowers blood pressure, blood sugar, stress, and is a great abdominal workout. Who doesn't like to laugh? The act of laughing and smiling releases serotonin in the brain, which makes us feel happy and relaxed. As serotonin increases, catecholamines (stress hormones) decrease.

Recent studies show that we don't laugh enough. I know life can seem too serious sometimes, so it can be helpful to intentionally work in some laugh time. For me, this may be listening to comedy radio during a workout, watching a light-hearted show, or just getting on the floor and making silly faces with my kids.

Have you ever noticed that after a child gets hurt, if you make them laugh, they instantly stop crying, jump up and resume play? That's because laughing can actually reduce pain symptoms. James Rotton, PH.D., of Florida International University, reported that post-surgical orthopedic patients who watched comedy shows while recovering, requested less pain medication than a control group that watched dramatic shows.

Do you laugh at least once a day? I'm not talking about a polite little chuckle. I mean a belly laugh, where you have to take a deep breath afterward. For most of us, the answer is probably no. How can we fix that?

Start by figuring out what makes you laugh. Is it a friend, a television show, or a funny video online? I can always depend on YouTube. I search for funny animals, but you can search for whatever tickles your funny bone.

Next, make a list of your top five laugh-makers. My list includes my family; my great friend, Lora; a comedy show; and comedy radio. It's great to have a few options to go between. I don't think Lora has time to crack me up every day, but we do aim for a chat at least once a week.

The next important factor is timing. Laughing is great anytime, but it can be especially helpful when you need to relax. Maybe your work environment could use a little lightening up. Post a funny joke in the breakroom or bathroom, and watch your coworker's moods change. Maybe you need to break the tension around the dinner table. Have a competition to see who can make the funniest joke. For me, I like to end my day with intentional laughter, so that's when I pull out my list and choose to do an activity that will make me laugh, brighten my soul, and help me relax. It's a great way to end the day and improve sleep.

Chapter 23
Helpful Hobbies

Do you like to create things? What did you enjoy doing as a child? Was it building puzzles, painting, sewing, scrapbooking, or working on cars? Everyone had something they enjoyed before the responsibilities of life intervened.

Remember coloring a picture? How did you feel about what you were doing? Were you thinking about how that coworker made you mad, or that deadline you needed to meet? Of course not. You were simply thinking about what color you wanted to use and if the picture was coming alive. When is the last time you thought about coloring?

My client, Susan, loved to paint as a child. She painted on canvas, plates, anything she could get ahold of. She could lose herself in this for hours, and always finished with a true feeling of accomplishment.

Hobbies can be incredibly satisfying. You simply put in the time and the productivity flows. There's no deadline or standards to meet. Thankfully, there no quality control. It's simply relaxing to spend time doing something you enjoy.

Besides the benefits of relaxing, decreasing stress levels, and creating a product that can be shared, there is another key advantage to indulging in a hobby. When we are busy with our hands, we are less tempted to put something in our mouths.

Imagine finishing dinner and daily chores, then plopping down in your favorite chair and turning on the TV. What normally happens next? For many of us, we get the urge to munch on something. That urge is your body telling you, "Hello! The stress of today was too much, and I need comfort. What are you going to do about it?"

So, we head to the kitchen in search of something to eat.

At first you might grab some crackers, but when that doesn't cut it, you head for the ice cream. After that, you're feeling guilty that you blew the whole day – especially when you were doing so well. Well, now that you've blown it, what's next...Oreos?

Have you been there? I know I have. It's like you have this weird, empty feeling that you try to fill with food, but the more food you put in it, the larger the hole gets. That's because your body is screaming out for comfort and relaxation. We tend to go for sweet, salty and starchy foods, because the excess carbohydrates cause our brains to release serotonin, giving us a (temporary) relaxed feeling.

Studies show that carbohydrates, especially sugar, react in our brain like crack cocaine. Food can literally be addicting, especially if you are stressed. As soon as the carbs start to digest, the hormones change and the body floods with insulin (the hormone to decrease blood sugar). As the blood sugar and insulin rise, the body leaves the comfort zone and moves to the stressed zone. Since you weren't even hungry when you ate that food, the body starts storing it as fat for later.

The extreme rise and crash in blood sugar keeps you in the stressed state for hours after that ice cream is long gone. It may even be the cause of your poor sleep at night. You wake up halfway through the night, unable to fall back asleep again. This is a classic sign that you are on the blood sugar roller coaster.

Susan knew all too well what I was talking about. Every evening after dinner, she would settle on the coach with a bowl of ice cream and bag of potato chips to watch her favorite TV drama. She had no idea that TV show was actually increasing her already sky high stress levels. After finishing the ice cream and chips, she would feel so bloated and tired that she would fall asleep on the coach - only to wake up at midnight and feel wide awake.

The lack of sleep would make work the next day seem impossible for Susan. She had no energy or drive to make her lunch or snacks after only sleeping for a few hours. And this pattern was repeated over and over again.

During a telephone session one morning, Susan could not stop yawning. She was trying to tell me about her food intake, but couldn't get through a sentence without yawning. This was my clue. I asked her how she was sleeping. "Horrible," she responded.

As we went through her daily food intake, I noticed she wasn't eating very much during the day.

"Well I'm trying so hard to lose weight and I'm not that hungry, so I just skip stuff. But then at night, I'm ravenous and eat everything in the kitchen. I feel so tired and guilty after, and I promise myself I won't ever do it again. But by the next evening, I feel so tired and stressed, that I do it again. I feel so embarrassed telling you this," Susan said.

I told Susan not to feel embarrassed, and that I knew exactly how she felt.

"But how can you? You probably eat super clean all the time," she responded.

I get that a lot, but the reality is I'm just like everyone else. I have stressful days and occasional cravings. It is freeing to know that the cravings are usually just our body's way of telling us it needs something. So what do you do when you can't shake the feeling, but the food isn't helping?

Often times, the stress of life can trigger that insatiable feeling to make unhealthy choices. The next time that happens, I encourage you stop and engage some mindful eating skills. What is your body telling you? Is your stomach growling, or do you feel hungry, shaky or weak? If the answer is no, you need something other than food.

Are you thirsty, tired or stressed? If so, drink some water, get some rest, or begin that hobby we have been talking about.

Susan made it her goal to work on this area. She felt so stressed and tired that she had been eating food to cope, but that was just making things worse. She decided to stop skipping meals and snacks, and to start painting for at least 30 minutes each evening.

After a few weeks, the weight started falling off. Susan was sleeping better after eating a handful of nuts and half an apple before bed. And sleeping for eight hours straight made her feel like superwoman, so planning and eating healthier choices became easier. She also felt less stressed during the day, and looked forward to painting each evening.

"I forgot how painting takes me away to a different world. I don't even think about work. I'm focused on blending the colors to get the perfect purple for the meadow of flowers I'm creating. Since I have one hand holding a brush and the other one holding the paint pallet, I'm not trying to eat my feelings. Instead, I paint how I feel. And I want to feel relaxed, so I purposely paint relaxing scenes," Susan shared.

A few months later, Susan was shopping for new clothes three sizes smaller. She also began taking painting classes. She even sent me the beautiful painting of the meadow with purple flowers.

Whatever you like to do or have enjoyed in the past, be like Susan and get back to it. Working on your hobby can improve your mood, and provide the comfort your body is asking for.

Chapter 24
Caring For Others Will Nourish Your Soul

Over the years, it has become abundantly clear that most of my clients are struggling with motivation. They find it hard to put in the time and effort it takes to care for themselves. This is a common human instinct that stems from the bigger picture. It is my belief that we are not on this earth to wander around aimlessly only caring for ourselves. It is important to care for ourselves, yes, but it is not the ultimate goal.

When you stop and think about why you want to lose weight and improve your health, odds are it is not just to look better. Most people want to feel better, too. They feel tired of being tired, overwhelmed, and undernourished. Most want to shed those unwanted pounds, because those pounds are holding them back from doing what they want in life - being contributing members in their families and communities. After all, does it really matter how nice we looked after we are gone? People will remember what we did in life, not just how we looked.

Bianca's story may be like yours. She is a mother, wife, and full-time purchasing agent that was too tired to be the mother, wife, and person she wanted to be. Before she had children, she used to go to the gym a few times a week. She had enough energy to survive in life, with a little extra for an occasional night out dancing with her husband. Her weight was not in great control, but she felt comfortable and had enough energy to get by.

After a promotion at work and having her handsome, energetic son, things changed. Bianca found herself barely able to make it to work and care for her family. Little things like laundry and housekeeping were completely overwhelming since she was so tired. But it wasn't a lack of energy for housekeeping that brought Bianca to me; it was the fact that she couldn't be an active mother.

Bianca's son would beg her to get on the ground and play with him, but every time she did, she could barely get up. He wanted to do things like play tag, but she couldn't chase him without gasping for breath.

"How did this happen? When I was in high school, I played on the soccer team and ran all day long in the heat. Sometimes even twice a day. How can a body go from that to this?" Bianca asked as she held back tears. "I just don't understand," she went on. "I know I need to change, but how can I change if I don't have the energy to try?"

During Bianca's session, we talked about how life would be different once she hit her goals. I asked her how losing 40 pounds would change things.

"Well," she took a deep breath and thought for a few minutes, "I think it would be a lot easier to play with my son if I wasn't carrying around all this extra weight. You don't understand how much of a workout it is just to get dressed, walk around at work, and then try to take care of my son. No wonder I don't have energy to do the fun stuff. I'm wasting it all on carrying around this stupid weight."

I asked Bianca how dropping the weight would change her relationship with her son.

"He would be so proud of me if I could play tag with him. Play baseball with him. Just get on the ground and be silly with him," she said.

Bianca started to cry when I asked her how she thought the changes would impact her son's life in the future.

"He would grow up knowing that his mother is happy and healthy. He would see how important it is to care for himself. If I don't change, he might grow up thinking that it isn't important to eat well – or he may end up like this tired, sad person I have become. I don't ever want him to feel like this! I want him to be healthy and have tons of energy, so he can do whatever he wants to do. I don't want his weight to hold him back, like my weight is doing to me," Bianca answered.

This was a powerful conversation. I could tell how badly Bianca wanted to change - so she could break the cycle and prevent her son from feeling how she felt.

Over the next few weeks, we modified Bianca's food intake to boost her energy and support a stable mood. We added a few supplements like a daily multivitamin, an energy boosting vitamin B Complex, and meal replacement shake options for when she didn't have time to cook.

Bianca used her Sundays to get organized. She prepped meals for the entire week, so after work all she had to do was heat and serve. As the nutrients started to replenish her deficiencies, her energy started to soar.

A few weeks later, Bianca shared her success.

"With more energy, I felt like it was time to give baseball another go for my son. Not only do I have the energy to take him to practice, but I actually volunteered to be a base coach. I'm standing, cheering, and running the whole time - and I don't even feel tired. He is so excited to have me out on the field playing with him. Shedding this weight is great, and I can fit better in my clothes. But the thing I am most excited about is that I am more present in my family's life. I'm not missing out anymore. I'm making memories to last a lifetime," said Bianca.

She continued, "And can you believe it? My picky son is actually eating vegetables now, because he sees me eating them. Not only is this helping me, but it is helping my whole family."

I was so happy for Bianca. Not only was she looking better, but more importantly she was feeling better. I asked her how her family life had changed, and it was such good news.

"I am finally enjoying life again, and so is my family. We are all so much happier now. I had no idea how my health was negatively affecting them. But now I see how important it is to take care of myself. Not just so I can feel better, but so I can give back to those I love. I want people to remember how much I loved and cared for them," Bianca shared.

Six months later, Bianca hit her goal weight and made a promise to care for herself so she can care for others.

"Caring for others feeds my soul. Seeing their faces light up because they know I care makes me happy." Well said, Bianca.

Chapter 25
Venture Outside

Humans are such unique creatures. We are so intelligent that we often forget about our physical health needs. We get tied up in work, or so bogged down in life, that we forget about the little things we need.

A great example of this is sunshine and fresh air. It is all too easy to get distracted by the life inside our phones and computers that we forget about the bigger picture. Have you ever been so mentally and emotionally consumed by a problem - maybe a deadline at work - that you can't think about anything else? I know I have been there; so immersed in a project that it becomes an unhealthy and imbalanced situation. It can easily start to feel like it's the most important thing the world.

That is why taking a break, and going for a walk outside can be so refreshing. Sometimes it takes the physical action of changing our environment to remember what life is all about. We are small stars shining in the sky of life. One action, or deadline, can make a difference, but it does not define us. Choices and actions can change our course if we allow them to control our future.

Getting outside can be a reminder that life is too short and too valuable to waste worrying about all the little things. After all, in five years, is that thing you are so worried about now even going to matter? A great friend once told me, "This, too, will pass."

This simple phrase can be a gentle reminder that all that seems crazy and overwhelming right now will pass in time. Sometimes we just need to ride the wave a little while until we can come out on the other side.

Have you ever stood at the seashore and just watched the waves? The ocean is so large and powerful, with the waves building up and crashing on the sand. And then, they are gone in an instant.

I challenge you to go out into nature and spend some time admiring how grand it all is. See how small we are compared to the vast size and power of Mother Nature. We are a very important part of this world, and there is not a single person out there just like us. We are completely unique, crafted in loving detail by our almighty creator.

You are here right now, in this exact position, for a specific purpose. What can you learn from this moment? What can you contribute to this moment? Mother Nature will nourish your soul if you allow her to. But we have to escape the confinements of our homes and offices to do so.

Another important reason to venture outside, is that we actually need sunlight and the vitamin D it provides. The vast majority of Americans are extremely deficient in the sunshine vitamin, and that increases our risk of developing cancer, diabetes, heart disease, depression, and more.

Vitamin D has been shown to boost our mood, provide energy, and protect against inflammatory diseases. If you haven't seen the sun in months, it's no wonder you feel tired and cranky.

Most of us live under roofs, drive to work in cars with UV protective windows, work in offices with fluorescent lighting, drive back home, and are so tired from work that we relax in front of the TV. We really don't see the light of day.

Light is such an important physical and spiritual component of life. Most life forms cannot survive without it, and we are no different. Sunlight not only nourishes our bodies, it nourishes our souls. When you close your eyes and think about a place that makes you feel happy, relaxed, and energized, what do you think of? Most likely you think of a place with light. For me, it's a serene beach with small waves rolling on shore, a light, warm breeze, and lots of sunshine.

Maybe for you, it's a hike on a trail surrounded by tall pine trees that smell so vibrant and fresh. Wherever it is, it is probably a place in the light of day.

Sunlight is a representation of energy and strength. It is a symbol of life, because without it, most things would not survive. We require it.

If you don't often see the light of day, it may be helpful to schedule in 20 to 30 minutes a day outside in the sunlight. This can be taking a walk, eating your lunch at a picnic table, or playing with the kids at the park. However you enjoy getting outside, make an effort to do it daily.

I normally aim for the mornings or evenings, when the UV rays are less intense. Even then, I sometimes prefer the indirect sunlight under the shade of a tree. Indirect light will still provide the necessary benefits of sunlight, but it's gentler on the body.

Even with daily sun exposure, it can be helpful to try and include more food products high in vitamin D. Some examples of these are fatty fish like tuna, mackerel, and salmon. Mushrooms, tofu, and eggs are also surprisingly high in vitamin D. Most dairy products, like milk and yogurt, are fortified with it.

Enjoying these foods in your daily intake is helpful, but recent studies show that our requirements are much higher than previously thought. It is very beneficial to add a vitamin D supplement to your daily regimen.

Between sunshine, food, and a little added help from a vitamin D supplement, we can boost our mood, and nourish our bodies and souls to feel better and protect against disease.

EPILOGUE

Thank you so much for the time we have shared together. I know this is a lot of information to digest, so take some time to step back for a minute and look at the big picture. Odds are you are here because you tried cutting out calories and were killing yourself at the gym, only to be disappointed in the results. But rest assured, it is most likely because you were missing a few key elements to a healthy, balanced nutritional intake and lifestyle.

The frustrating thing is, that if any part of your mind, body or soul is out of whack, the whole system can get off kilter and send you into a downward spiral. Bringing all three back into balance is vital to obtaining your goals.

May you feel relieved to know that there is hope. You do deserve to look and feel your best, and it might be easier than you think. When you are deep in the knowledge of these pages, it might seem overwhelming to put it all together. Once you read through the book, it can be helpful to go back and use the chapters as a checklist. Start from the beginning and check off the chapters you already feel you are successful at in your life.

Maybe your soul is rich and nourished, but your mind needs a boost in its belief in your personal success. Maybe you have read every self-help book out there, and already believe deep in your heart and mind that you will succeed, but you need the exact nutrition knowledge to be your road map.

If you are like many of the wonderful people I help, perhaps your life recipe just needs a little spicing up. Most of us need a pinch of personal belief, a dash of nutritional knowledge, and a heaping dose of spirit to achieve success. Combining these ingredients in the right measurements will launch you toward your goal of losing weight, by nurturing your mind, body, and soul.

Just like any recipe that you personalize, you may need to adjust an ingredient here and there until you find the perfect combination. You will know you've got it right when you start shedding those pounds, and feel your body come back into balance. It may take a few weeks, and for some, even a few months, but stick with it.

Years of research and application has gone into creating this recipe for success. I am here to help you every step along the way through my personalized nutritional coaching program.

For more information, visit me online at ThriveNutritionandFitness.com. My team and I offer personalized nutritional coaching, group nutrition classes, personal training, group fitness classes, yoga, and more.

RESOURCES

"The Hormone Cure" by Sara Gottfried, M.D.

"Why Am I Still Fat?" by Dietitian Cassie, R.D.

American Sleep Association

Thrive Nutrition & Fitness

Nutrition and fitness coaching provides the best results. To schedule your session, visit www.ThriveNutritionandFitness.com.

Services: Individual Nutritional Coaching; Group Nutritional Coaching; Group Fitness Instruction; Personal Training; and more...

About Nicole Gilles

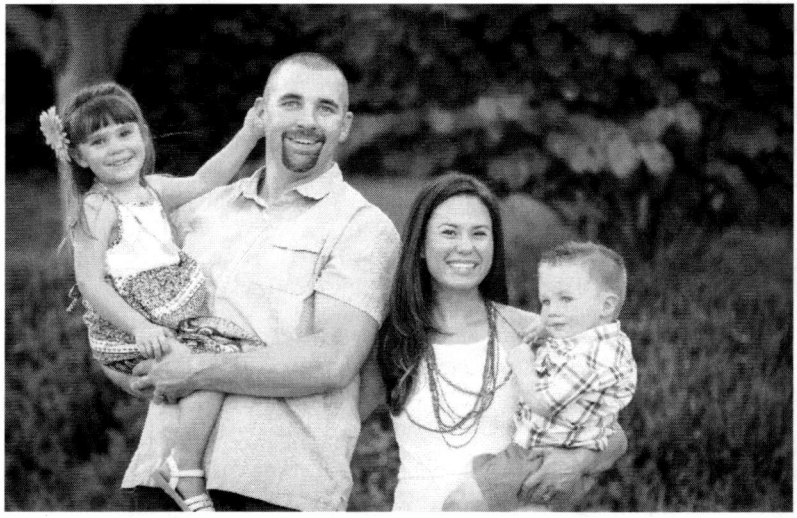

Nicole Gilles is a Registered Dietitian who specializes in Weight Management. She is Board Certified in Adult Weight Management, Diabetes, and Kidney Nutrition. But since weight loss is about more than just eating well and exercising, Nicole has gone a step further to specialize in Hormone Therapy. If hormones are unbalanced, it can slow or prevent weight loss, and effect emotional and mental health.

As a mother of two young children, Nicole understands what it takes to eat well and stay active. This can feel like an impossible task when you feel like life has taken your time and energy hostage. But with a little planning, it can become easy.

Nicole's passion is not just promoting healthy weight loss and maintenance, but sharing how nutrition and exercise can give you more energy, strength, and joy. Join her on her journey to share the gift of good health and well-being.